EMOTION IN THERAPY

Also by Stefan G. Hofmann

Treating Chronic and Severe Mental Disorders:
A Handbook of Empirically Supported Interventions
Edited by Stefan G. Hofmann and Martha C. Tompson

Emotion in Therapy

From Science to Practice

Stefan G. Hofmann

Foreword by Steven C. Hayes

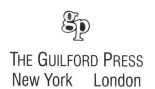

THE GUILFORD PRESS
New York   London

The author has checked with sources believed to be reliable in his efforts to provide information
that is complete and generally in accord with the standards of practice that are accepted at the time
of publication. However, in view of the possibility of human error or changes in behavioral, mental
health, or medical sciences, neither the author, nor the editors and publisher, nor any other party
who has been involved in the preparation or publication of this work warrants that the information
contained herein is in every respect accurate or complete, and they are not responsible for any errors
or omissions or the results obtained from the use of such information. Readers are encouraged to
confirm the information contained in this book with other sources.

Library of Congress Cataloging-in-Publication Data

Hofmann, Stefan G.
  Emotion in therapy : from science to practice / Stefan G. Hofmann ; foreword by
Steven C. Hayes.— First Edition.
     pages cm
  Includes bibliographical references and index.
  ISBN 978-1-4625-2448-8 (hardback : alk. paper)
  1. Emotions. 2. Emotion-focused therapy. I. Title.
  BF531.H64 2016
  152.4—dc23
                                                                    2015031049

To Rosemary, Benjamin, and Lukas

About the Author

Stefan G. Hofmann, PhD, is Professor of Psychology in the Department of Psychological and Brain Sciences at Boston University, where he directs the Psychotherapy and Emotion Research Laboratory. He has an actively funded research program studying various aspects of emotional disorders, with a particular emphasis on anxiety disorders and cognitive-behavioral therapy (CBT). Dr. Hofmann is the recipient of many prestigious professional awards, including the 2015 Aaron T. Beck Award from the Academy of Cognitive Therapy and the 2012 Aaron T. Beck Award for Excellence in Contributions to CBT from the Institute for Cognitive Studies at Assumption College; he has also been named a Highly Cited Researcher by Thomson Reuters. He is a Fellow of the American Psychological Association and the Association for Psychological Science and is past president of numerous national and international professional societies, including the Association for Behavioral and Cognitive Therapies and the International Association for Cognitive Psychotherapy. Dr. Hofmann is the editor in chief of *Cognitive Therapy and Research* and has published 15 books, including *An Introduction to Modern CBT: Psychological Solutions to Mental Health Problems*, and more than 300 peer-reviewed journal articles. For more information, visit *www.bostonanxiety.org*.

Foreword

It would be hard to choose a topic that is more talked about but yet is harder to get a grasp on than emotion. Almost every case consultation, case conference, or clinical hour will include emotional terms— lots of them. Emotional labels are used often to name or describe clinical disorders. Clients explain their needs and wants using them. If you put a reasonable sample of emotional terms into websites such as *Google Books Ngram Viewer* or *WordNet–Affect*, you will quickly realize that hardly anything substantial exists in the English literature that does not in some way touch emotional experience.

There is a reason for this extensive use: felt and expressed emotion does a huge amount of work for human beings. It tells us things about our bodies, our history, and our predispositions. It helps us to understand ourselves, to predict our own actions, and to tell others what we need or want. And that is just a start.

In this important new book, Stefan G. Hofmann summarizes the vast literature on emotion and links it to clinical practice. He does it in a style that I think is particularly useful, and I want to direct the readers' attention to that style so that they are more likely to benefit from it.

You can sense what a task Hofmann has set for himself as soon as *emotion* is defined in the first pages of Chapter 1.

An emotion is (1) a multidimensional experience that is (2) characterized by different levels of arousal and degrees of pleasure–displeasure; (3) associated with subjective experiences, somatic sensations, and motivational tendencies; (4) colored by contextual and culture factors; and that (5) can be regulated to some degree through intra- and interpersonal processes. (p. 2)

This definition involves key topics in psychology such as

- Experience
- Physiological arousal
- Sensation
- Motivation
- Culture
- Context—encompassing both history and circumstance
- The valence of experience
- Self-regulation
- Social regulation

The list is daunting, but it would be a deep error to let the length of the list stop us in our tracks. Emotional experience is too central to human experience to be put aside merely because it is complicated or is not easy to define and to measure.

Hofmann understands that emotion is a kind of node in a large network of topics. This book explores that network; it fills it out. It does not force the node into a neat and tidy little box: anxiety is "really" this, or sadness is "really" that. Emotion is just not that easily packaged; it's inherently multidimensional and multifaceted. This is exactly why many lesser authors have avoided doing a deep dive into the topic but also why this particular book is so useful, and why I think the approach this book takes to the topic is so wise.

In applied psychological work we see a lot of extremes in the treatment of emotion: emotional experience is the central topic and an area of concern for all clinical work; emotion is important, but only as a kind of side effect of other processes (e.g., cognition); emotion is an epiphenomenon; emotion is merely a social construction; emotion is nothing but bodily sensations and behavioral predispositions. There are entire systems of psychotherapy that barely mention emotion and others that have a hard time mentioning anything else.

These theorists plant a flag in one part of the array of issues engaged by emotion, but at the cost of considering and appreciating the whole of it.

This book manages never to fall into any of these extremes because it has another purpose: to empower the reader to address the topic from multiple angles. It wants the reader to see the network itself, not just one node within that network. It brings a seriousness of thought and a healthy dose of skepticism to the topic, at the same time that it maintains its fascination with emotion and a foundational sense of deep importance. It invites the reader into that same posture of openness, seriousness, curiosity, and caring that helps clinicians and researchers alike maintain a balanced perspective when considering how emotion can be of applied use.

You will not leave this volume with a single view of emotion forced down your throat. You will leave instead with an appreciation for the many facets of this domain and with clinical and research avenues to explore. That is a kind of intellectual and practical empowerment that is unusual and is deeply respectful of the reader. You will never be talked down to, you will never be abandoned, and you will never be bullied. Instead there is a sense of the systematic use of science and reason to dismantle and examine a critically important topic that every psychotherapist and every school of psychological thought needs to confront. The book will guide and help, but it will not dictate.

Each of the chapters ends with a summary that extends what you have read into a set of short points that can be used to guide clinical practice. I strongly suggest that you give these summaries a lot of attention. They are not merely mechanical summaries: they are nuggets. You could do a lot of good just by reviewing them before sessions because they synthesize so much.

Let me give a few quick examples. Here are three statements drawn from summaries in different parts of the book.

- "In order to gain further clarity about their emotional states, patients may be instructed to explore not only their thoughts and feelings about specific events or triggers, but also their thoughts and feelings about their initial/primary feelings." (p. 23)

- "Emotion regulation strategies per se are neither good nor bad. Rather, effectiveness depends on the adaptiveness of an emotion regulation strategy to the particular situational demand and goal achievement." (p. 102)
- "People tend to overestimate the intensity of positive and negative affect they think they will experience if a particular event happens because people underestimate the importance of self-regulatory processes and because people tend not to consider the surrounding circumstances that will co-occur with that event in the future (which is known as focalism)." (p. 82)

There is a great deal of wisdom here, and by the time you read these points they will have become useful clinical hooks for an entire network of knowledge. There are dozens of short points of this kind in the book, and the knowledge behind them will subtly change how you think about the entire topic of emotion in a way that gives both practitioners and researchers useful paths to explore.

That is an enormous service to the field. This book is an unusual contribution that should be appreciated, savored—and then used.

STEVEN C. HAYES, PHD
Foundation Professor of Psychology
University of Nevada, Reno

Acknowledgments

A popular Chinese proverb and the content of one of my fortune cookies reads: *A journey of a thousand miles must begin with a single step*. This page is the last step after a long journey that took many steps. I am glad that I did not know how long a journey it would be after taking the first step, because some of the parts were much more difficult than I had first anticipated. I spent countless hours writing, rewriting, organizing, and reorganizing the text and even more time reading, researching, and simply thinking about the issues. Some of these ideas took long enough to work out to yield a number of published journal articles. At various points, I felt that I might have bitten off much more than I could chew. Instead of giving up or settling for less, I started chewing more slowly.

Writing this book meant taking time away from my family. Thanks to my wife, Rosemary, and my sons, Benjamin and Lukas, for allowing me to do what I needed to do. I could not have done it without your support. Also, many thanks to Jim Nageotte, Senior Editor at The Guilford Press, for his patience and guidance. It was clear that Jim and I shared the same goal, and we did not want to settle for less.

My students are a constant source of inspiration. Thanks to Anu Asnaani, Joseph Carpenter, Joshua Curtiss, Angela Fang, Cassidy Gutner, Shelley Kind, and Ty Sawyer. You are among the main reasons why I am convinced that I have the best job in the world. Also, many thanks to my mentors and friends. There are too many to name them all, but I am especially grateful to David Barlow, Anke Ehlers, Aaron T. Beck, and Steven Hayes. For some brief moments, I was standing on the shoulders of giants and wondering how I got there.

The journey has ended now, and what a long, strange trip it's been. As is true for many exciting trips, I enjoyed the ride most of the time, but I am also glad that I finally arrived at my destination. The journey taught me a lot, and I hope I was able to share what I have learned about improving emotional health.

Preface

The purpose of this book is to translate insights from emotion research into clinical applications. Emotions are key determinants of mental health. The ability to deal successfully with emotions is an important human characteristic that facilitates social adjustment and overall well-being. Pursuing important life goals requires tolerance and management of a wide range of affective states, including uncomfortable and distressing feelings. Ineffective strategies for dealing with emotions are the central source of many psychological problems. In fact, the vast majority of psychological problems are emotional problems. Some of these problems can be effectively treated with psychological interventions, such as cognitive-behavioral therapy (CBT). Although many people improve after these treatments, they are often far from being healthy and happy human beings free of emotional distress. Treatments that move beyond the level of illness symptoms can significantly improve their personal emotional health and quality of life. In this book, I present several approaches not only to reducing suffering but also to achieving improved well-being by translating findings from emotion and motivation research, affective science, and social psychology into clinical practice.

Despite how central emotions are to mental health, there are few concrete clinical recommendations for dealing with emotions specifically. To illustrate how the research can be translated into specific clinical techniques, in each chapter I present sections labeled as "In Practice," together with case illustrations and closing summaries to highlight some of the clinically relevant information discussed in the chapter.

Recent studies suggest that specific strategies to enhance emotional health can, in fact, enhance existing treatments for mental disorders. It has further been shown that individuals differ in their habitual ways of managing their emotions and that those individual differences are meaningfully associated with psychosocial functioning. For example, it has been found that individuals who habitually use reappraisal to regulate emotions experience more positive emotion and less negative emotion overall, have better interpersonal functioning, and report greater well-being. In contrast, individuals who habitually use suppression experience less positive emotion and greater negative emotion, have worse interpersonal functioning, and report lower well-being. Moreover, it appears that any specific emotion regulation strategy, in itself, is neither adaptive nor maladaptive. Rather, it is the context and situational demands that determine whether a particular strategy is adaptive. Therefore, ideally we should develop the ability to flexibly apply any particular strategy in order to achieve the desirable goals and avoid undesirable outcomes.

It is important to note, however, that this book is not merely focused on emotion regulation. The term *emotion regulation* has become a relatively narrow research topic in social psychology with (in my view) relatively limited relevance to clinical practice. The term *emotion*, on the other hand, is broad and complicated. My primary objective, as I have noted, is to translate the knowledge acquired from various disciplines examining emotions into formulating concrete clinical strategies, with the goal of enhancing psychotherapy for a variety of psychological problems. The disciplines I review include affective neuroscience, laboratory-based emotion research, biology, anthropology, social and personality research, psychiatry, and even Buddhist and other religious practices.

The strategies that I describe are *transdiagnostic*. Although the empirical evidence aligns them most closely to CBT, they are not confined to any particular psychotherapy model. They offer clinicians concrete recommendations for incorporating emotions into traditional psychosocial treatments. The book contains eight chapters, briefly summarized as follows. Chapter 1 discusses the nature of emotions and reviews the most influential and relevant emotion theories. Chapter 2 identifies individual differences as they relate to the experience, expression, and regulation of emotions. Emotions are directly associated with approach and avoidance tendencies and goal attainment. Therefore, Chapter 3 discusses the relationship between motivation and emotion. Chapter 4 reviews the self and self-regulation as applied to emotions, and Chapter 5 examines in detail one such self-regulation strategy: emotion regulation. Chapter 6 is dedicated to appraisal and reappraisal, important aspects of CBT. Chapter 7 discusses mindfulness and meditation strategies, including loving-kindness meditation, for enhancing positive affect, a generally neglected but important aspect of emotional health. Finally, Chapter 8 provides a brief overview of the neurobiological correlates of emotions and emotion regulation.

The readership I had in mind when writing this book consists of clinicians and health care professionals interested in the newest and cutting-edge psychological treatment approaches. I learned a lot when researching this fascinating field and enjoyed summarizing and translating it to derive concrete treatment strategies. I hope I have succeeded.

Contents

Purchasers of this book can download and
print enlarged versions of select figures at
www.guilford.com/hofmann3-forms for
personal use or use with individual clients
(see copyright page for details).

CHAPTER ONE

◆

The Nature of Emotions

The ability to experience emotions is an essential human quality. Lieutenant Commander Data, one of the characters in the popular TV series *Star Trek: The Next Generation,* was a human-looking robot (android) who showed all but one human trait: He lacked the ability to experience emotions. In many episodes, this inability was portrayed as the quintessential missing piece of being fully human. Despite his intelligence, it was difficult for Data to understand (and for his human colleagues to explain) the nature of emotions. At one point, Data's character dramatically changed when an emotion chip was implanted into his positronic network in the *Star Trek* movie *Brothers.* He then transformed from an intelligent and self-aware machine into a human being.

But what exactly is an emotion? What are its defining characteristics? What is the difference between an emotion and affect? What is the relationship between thoughts and emotions? Do emotions serve a purpose and a function? How are emotions experienced, how are they created, and how do they relate to behaviors and mental illnesses?

These are the questions I tackle in this chapter. Spoiler alert:

There is no one-sentence definition; an emotion is a multidimensional and multilayered construct, and there are many related terms that are used to define an emotion.

DEFINING EMOTION

For starters, the working definition of emotion used in this book is the following:

An emotion is (1) a multidimensional experience that is (2) characterized by different levels of arousal and degrees of pleasure–displeasure; (3) associated with subjective experiences, somatic sensations, and motivational tendencies; (4) colored by contextual and cultural factors; and that (5) can be regulated to some degree through intra- and interpersonal processes.

This definition implies that emotions include biological systems that are often (but not necessarily) associated with evolutionary adaptations and motivational tendencies and that are shaped by social, cultural, and other contextual factors. A brief review of the contemporary neurobiological basis of emotions is given in Chapter 8.

An emotion is an experience. So when we *have an emotion,* we refer to the *experience* of an emotion. This experience is typically (but not always) elicited by a stimulus, such as a situation, an event, another person, a thought, or a memory. Most of the time (but again, not always), we are aware of this experience and aware of the stimulus that triggered it. In Chapter 8, I examine in more detail the different levels of (conscious and unconscious) processing of emotional material.

The *emotional experience* and the *emotional response* are functionally linked. Simply put, the term *emotional response* refers to reacting to emotion-eliciting stimuli or triggers, whereas the term *emotional experience* refers to linking a label to this response. As discussed in more detail later in the chapter, William James (1884) and Carl Lange (1887) considered an emotion to be merely the feeling of specific bodily responses to a situation. This theory became known as the James–Lange theory of emotions. Later cognitively oriented emotion theorists assume that an emotional experience is the result of the cognitive appraisal of a general physiological arousal (Schachter & Singer, 1962).

Emotions per se are neither *bad* nor *good* but are often experienced as pleasant or unpleasant, depending on contextual factors such as specific situational aspects and the person's interpretations of them. The definition further suggests that emotions can be regulated to some extent, both intrapersonally through cognitive strategies, such as reappraisal or suppression, and interpersonally through other people. Moreover, emotions are rarely pure but are "messy" experiences. They are typically experienced as mixtures and blends of various emotions (e.g., being happy and sad, angry and fearful), and different emotions can be linked to form complex networks, resulting in emotions about emotions (a notion that I discuss in more detail later).

Definitions of emotion vary depending on whether one adopts a nature or a nurture perspective (i.e., whether one assumes emotions are biologically hardwired versus seeing them as a product of the social context). The definition I use includes both a nature component and a nurture aspect; emotions are shaped by context and cognitions, but they also have a clear biological and evolutionary basis. More than a decade after his major contribution on evolution that would revolutionize the field of science, Darwin wrote *The Expression of Emotions in Man and Animals* (1872/1955), in which he discussed the evolutionary significance of emotions. In this book, Darwin makes the case that emotional expressions are universal across different ages and even species. He observed:

> The movements of expression in the face and body . . . serve as the first means of communication between the mother and her infant; she smiles approval, and thus encourages her child on the right path, or frowns disapproval. We readily perceive sympathy in others by their expression; our sufferings are thus mitigated and our pleasures increased; and mutual good feeling is thus strengthened. The movements of expression give vividness and energy to our spoken words. They reveal the thoughts and intentions of others more truly than do words, which may be falsified. (p. 364)

Darwin assigns emotions an important communicative function and closely ties emotions to cognitions. Cognitions, in turn, also serve an important evolutionary function because they allow the organism to predict, based on limited information, whether a situation is likely to lead to a desirable versus an undesirable state. Depending on this prediction, the organism then makes a decision to behave in a way that maximizes the likelihood of achieving the pleasurable state or avoiding the undesirable state. Cognitions and emotions closely interact with behaviors in a complex process that includes sensory input, attention, and information stored in long-term and short-term memory. Similar to anatomical structures, this process is assumed to have evolved to form adaptive structures that serve to increase evolutionary fitness for the individual.

BASIC EMOTIONS

Influenced by Darwin's view, a number of theorists have proposed that emotions are based on biological systems that have evolved to govern behaviors and to promote survival of the species, including the human race (e.g., Tomkins, 1963, 1982; Ekman, 1992a; Izard, 1992). These and other theorists have postulated the existence of a set of *basic* emotions that are likely to be found in all human cultures and that share similarities with different species. This set of basic emotions is assumed to fulfill useful, evolutionarily adaptive functions in dealing with fundamental life tasks by mobilizing quick and adaptive reactions in response to environmental changes. Thus, basic emotions are conceived as evolutionarily adaptive responses to situational demands. Ekman (1992a) posits that a feeling constitutes a basic emotion if (1) it has a quick onset; (2) it is of brief duration; (3) it occurs involuntarily; (4) the autonomic appraisal of the event that triggers it leads to an almost instant recognition of the stimulus; (5) its antecedent events are universal (i.e., are not specific to one particular culture); (6) the feeling is accompanied by a unique pattern of physiological symptoms; and (7) it is characterized by distinctive universal signals in the form of singular facial expressions and behavior.

This definition is closely aligned with a Darwinian perspective of emotion as a biologically based and evolutionarily adaptive response to environmental stimuli. Such basic emotions, which are found in virtually all human cultures (i.e., are universal), include happiness, sadness, fear, anger, and disgust/contempt and are expressed in unique facial expressions (Ekman, Friesen, & Ellsworth, 1972). The advantage of such a conceptualization lies in its simplicity, which allows for experimental testing by measuring, for example, people's physiological responses and facial expressions to discrete stimuli. As a result, many investigators have examined emotions in the laboratory as a linear input-out regulatory mechanism. This has led to a large number of laboratory-based experimental studies of emotion and emotion regulation (which are reviewed in Chapters 5 and 6). At the same time, this conceptualization ignores many complexities of human emotions, such as individual differences in the emotional experience, motivational tendencies associated with emotions, interpersonal and contextual factors that shape the experience and the expressions of emotions, and the meta-experience of emotions (i.e., emotions about emotions), all of which are discussed throughout this book.

The *basic emotion* concept was challenged soon after it was introduced (e.g., Ortony & Turner, 1990), and the challenge was rebutted (Ekman, 1992b). Similarly, Plutchik (1980) assumed existence of a set of basic emotions. More specifically, he proposed, similar to the color wheel, a circumplex model that includes a set of eight basic bipolar emotions: *joy* versus *sorrow, anger* versus *fear, acceptance* versus *disgust,* and *surprise* versus *expectancy.* All human emotions are assumed to result from a mixture of these eight basic emotions, similar to how we create a wide spectrum from mixing the three primary colors. For example, within this circumplex model, it is assumed that love includes elements of joy and acceptance.

Related to basic emotions are primary emotion processes (Panksepp & Biven, 2010), or biologically hardwired and evolutionarily older systems (i.e., systems that evolved early in the process of evolution). These systems include the *fear system,* which allows the organism to reflexively withdraw, hide, or run away; the *grief* (or separation-distress, formerly called *panic*) *system,* active when the organism experiences loss, which is associated with bereavement and mourning; the *rage system,* which is active during acts of aggression; the *seeking system,* which is active when the organism is searching for food or sexual partners; the *lust system,* which is active during sexual acts; the *care system,* which is active when raising offspring;

and the *play system,* which is active when playing with offspring, as well as when we are developing social skills. These different systems can be coactivated and work synergistically. For example, the *panic system* in conjunction with the *care system* leads to social bonding and social attachment.

CHARACTERISTICS OF EMOTIONS

Emotional experiences are complex and differ on many levels. Some emotions are strong, others are weak; some are pleasant, others unpleasant; some are short and others long lasting; some emotions are clear and raw, others are complicated and complex; some emotions feel under our control, others feel overwhelming and out of our control; and some emotions are associated with a strong urge to act, whereas others immobilize us. Despite the wide range of different emotional experiences, it is believed that there are laws that govern all emotions.

General Laws

Frijda (1988) described a number of these general laws (12 in total). First, an emotion depends on the interpretation of the situation. This law has been referred to as the *law of situational meaning.* This is a simple but critical observation that I discuss in more detail in the next section. In addition, one could argue that the interpretation is not limited to the situation but also to the experience associated with the emotion. Again, this observation is discussed in more detail later.

Second, the emotional experience depends on the person's subjective goals, motives, and concerns. This law has been referred to as the *law of concern.* We are happy when we win one of the many rounds of golf we play on Sunday mornings, whereas we are ecstatic if we win an important and long-anticipated tournament. Third, emotional experiences increase in intensity as the degree of reality increases (the *law of apparent reality).* Therefore, the feeling of joy after winning a miniature golf game against one's spouse is experienced as less intense than the winning of a tournament against Tiger Woods.

Emotions are elicited less by the presence of desirable or undesirable conditions than by the actual or expected *changes* in desirable or undesirable conditions (the fourth, fifth, and sixth laws: the *laws of change, habituation,* and *comparative feeling*). Therefore, the emotion one experiences when sinking a jump shot to win a regular-season game is experienced as more intense than the emotion associated with having won last year's game.

The seventh law (the *law of hedonic asymmetry*) states that continued pleasure (and displeasure) eventually wears off because the intensity of an emotion depends on the reference framework of the event that elicited the emotion. Therefore, somebody will experience a much greater degree of joy right after winning a million dollars in a lottery than days, months, and years later.

Without repeated exposure to the emotional events, emotions tend to be conserved (the eighth law: the *law of conservation of emotional momentum*). Therefore, avoiding dealing with a traumatic memory can lead to the conservation (i.e., maintenance and persistence) of the emotions associated with the trauma.

The ninth law (the *law of closure*) states that an emotional experience is perceived as being unique and absolute. For example, it seems impossible to love two different people exactly the same way and to the same degree. Although we feel absolute and unconditional love toward all of our children, those of us who are parents will admit that we love them slightly differently and for different reasons (and some even more than others). On the other hand, however, emotions are rarely experienced as pure, unequivocal, and absolute. Most of the time, emotional experiences are complex and multifaceted. For example, we might admire, fear, love, and hate our parents, and this mixture of emotions will change throughout our upbringing.

Responses associated with emotions are often complex because we tend to modify them based on the possible consequences these impulses might have (the tenth law: the *law of care of consequences*). We also tend to perceive ambiguous emotional events in such a way as to minimize the degree to which the events are painful or hard to endure (i.e., we tend to minimize the negative emotional load). At the same time, we perceive ambiguous situations in a way that maximizes our emotional gain. These two laws have been described as the *law of the lightest load* (the eleventh law) and the *law of the greatest gain* (the twelfth law).

The Transient Nature of Emotions

Regardless of the complexity of an emotion, it varies with time. We might fall in love with somebody and feel overwhelming joy. As time progresses and we realize the many difficulties the relationship brings, the emotional experience might change into sadness, despair, or a sense of loss. These feelings might mix and make us feel torn, with an urge to act upon them in contradictory ways. Part of us might want to approach, and the other part might want to avoid and even push away, the very person we feel attracted to.

Some emotional experiences occur over a period of seconds, such as surprise, whereas others (such as love) can last years or a lifetime. Obviously, it could be argued that love is not an emotional state but rather a general approach and perspective toward something or somebody. This is different from a short-lived and circumscribed emotional experience, such as surprise or fear. The more diffuse and far-reaching experience of love is more comparable to a trait or disposition to feel a particular (positive) way toward something or someone given a particular context. For example, a loving father is more likely to experience joy toward his child when he hears him practice the violin, whereas a tired neighbor may be irritated and angered by the violin lesson.

Cognitions and Emotions

The characteristics of emotional experiences highlight the importance of the reference framework in which these emotions are experienced, the situational context, and, most important, cognitive appraisals. Consider the following insights by some great thinkers: "People are not moved by things, but the view they take of them" (the Greek Stoic philosopher Epictetus, 55–134 C.E.); "If you are distressed by anything external, the pain is not due to the thing itself, but to your estimate of it, and this you have the power to revoke at any moment" (the Roman emperor Marcus Aurelius, 121–180 C.E.); and "There is nothing either good or bad, but thinking makes it so" (the playwright William Shakespeare, in *Hamlet*).

These insights can be reduced to the simple proposition that situations, events, or triggers do not directly cause an emotional response but that it is the cognitive appraisal of the situation, event, or trigger that leads to the emotional response. In other words, it is not the triggers that make us angry, anxious, happy, or sad, but it is the interpretation of the triggers. Therefore, it is important to identify the thought that is related to an emotion.

Although thoughts often lead to emotions, thoughts and emotions (as well as behaviors) do not stand in a unidirectional (one-way) relationship. Emotions can also affect thoughts when people use emotions to make sense of what is happening around them. For example, feeling high anxiety when waiting for one's spouse to come home can make the person think that "something terrible *must* have happened." Human brains are hardwired to take threatening information seriously, because ignoring it could endanger our survival. Similar relationships between thoughts and feelings exist for other emotions, such as sadness, anger, and so forth.

Thinking and reasoning often happen on an automatic level. Monitoring and observing one's thoughts can slow the process down and provide an opportunity to study the nature of one's thoughts. Meditation strategies, which are covered in Chapter 7, encourage present-moment awareness. These strategies interrupt automatic tendencies and intensify positive experiences.

Thoughts are not facts, but rather they are "hypotheses" that may or may not be correct. Some hypotheses (thoughts) are more probable than others (e.g., "my coughing is a sign of lung cancer" vs. "I have a cold"); other thoughts are almost certainly inaccurate ("tomorrow the world will end"); yet other thoughts are correct but are maladaptive ("I am going to die, we are all going to die, and the world will cease to exist"). No matter what thoughts we tend to have, it is important to bring them into awareness in order to evaluate their validity, probability adaptiveness, and so forth.

Throughout the history of psychology, different theories have been proposed to explain the relationship between cognitions and emotions and specifically the sequence of events and the direction of causality. The James–Lange theory of emotions posits that situational stimuli trigger specific and unique physiological responses, such as an increase in heart rate and respiration. At the same time, we show a particular behavior in response to the situation, such as withdrawal behaviors. Once we become aware of this unique pattern of somatovisceral arousal, we label this experience as "fear" after the initial response to the event occurred. Thus different emotional experiences are thought to arise because specific physiological symptoms and behaviors are linked to these emotional experiences. For example, the theory states that we experience fear because threatening situations lead to specific physiological symptoms (e.g., rapid heart rate and breathing rate) and behaviors (e.g., we startle or escape). Consistent with this theory are studies of people with spinal cord injuries showing that individuals with damage high on the spinal cord (quadriplegia) experience emotions as less intense than those with low injury (paraplegia). The theory can explain this phenomenon because an injury high on the spinal cord cuts off sensory feedback from a greater portion of the body (Hohmann, 1966).

However, there are also significant and obvious weaknesses associated with the James–Lange theory. For example, the theory assumes that subtle differences in sensory feedback distinguish among the wide variety of emotional experiences. However, psychophysiological studies have been unable to identify clear biological markers or unique physiological correlates to emotional states. Furthermore, simply inducing physiological arousal (e.g., by doing physical exercise) does not lead to emotional experience, and the physiological arousal is in many cases too slow and too general to account for the latency and variety of emotional expressions.

Based on these and other criticisms, Cannon (1927) and Bard (1934) formulated a competing theory suggesting that undifferentiated physiological arousal, such as the fight-or-flight response, triggers the emotion. According to the Cannon–Bard theory, the thalamus channels sensory input to the cerebral cortex and also sends activation messages through the autonomic nervous system to the viscera and skeletal muscles.

The influential theory and groundbreaking experiments by Schachter and Singer (1962) highlight the crucial importance of the cognitive processes in emotions. Consistent with Festinger's (1954) theory, it is assumed that a state of arousal prompts a desire by the individual to account for the perceived activation. Thus, a person who experiences a general and undifferentiated state of heightened arousal experiences a need to evaluate and interpret this arousal by using situation clues.

This theory posits that the intensity of an emotion is determined by the physiological arousal, whereas the valence and quality of the emotional response is determined by the appraisal of the triggering stimulus and context. In contrast to the James–Lange theory, the Schachter–Singer model does not assume that any physiological symptoms are specific or unique to any emotional experience. Instead, it is assumed that the same general physiological arousal can be interpreted in different ways, depending on the appraisal (i.e., interpretation) of the eliciting stimuli.

This model is best illustrated in the classic 1962 experiment by Schachter and Singer. In this study, participants were deceived and told they would be participating in an experiment on the effects of vitamins on vision. Instead, participants received either epinephrine or a placebo. Epinephrine is the synthetic form of adrenaline and temporarily increases heart and respiration rate and blood pressure and causes muscle tremors and a jittery feeling. Participants were then randomly assigned to different groups based on information about the effect of the injection and also based on the situational context. One group of participants received accurate information about the physiological effects of the injection (informed group); a second group was given no information about any physiological effects of the substance (uninformed group); and a third group received inaccurate information (misinformed group). Half of the participants from each of these groups were then assigned to different situational contexts, which consisted of one of two staged social interactions between a confederate and the participant. In one of the two conditions, participants were exposed to a euphoria condition in which the confederate behaved in a happy manner, engaging in such playful activity as shooting baskets by throwing paper wads into a trash can. In the other condition, participants were assigned to an anger condition in which the confederate clearly expressed his anger about the experiment, tearing up a questionnaire and eventually storming out of the room. The participants' behaviors were observed through a one-way mirror and rated by independent judges. Participants were also asked about their emotional states.

The results showed that participants in the informed group did not report any strong emotion, because they attributed their physiological arousal to the injection. In contrast, participants in the uninformed and misinformed groups did not have an obvious explanation for the physiological arousal induced by the injection. They therefore relied on the experimental situation and the confederates' behavior to interpret and label the physiological arousal they were experiencing. This study points to the importance of cognitive variables to emotions and shows that it is the appraisal of the physiological arousal, rather than the arousal itself, that determines the emotional experience. The Schachter and Singer cognitive appraisal model of emotions is consistent with many other observations and earlier theorists, ranging as far back as Epictetus (135 C.E./2013). However, this model is unlikely to account for every emotional experience. It is especially difficult to apply this theory to sudden emotional experiences that occur immediately following an event, such as the fear that one might experience after a near car accident. Therefore, modern theories of emotions assume that cognitions are involved at the outset of an emotional experience to varying degrees, depending on the time point of the emotional process.

AFFECT VERSUS EMOTION

The two terms *affect* and *emotion* are closely related constructs and are often used interchangeably. However, for the purpose of our discussion, I use these two terms separately. Consistent with other authors (e.g., Barrett, Mesquita, Ochsner, & Gross, 2007), I suggest that the term *affect* is used to describe the *subjective experience* of an emotional state that defines the valence of it. At its core, affect is experienced as positive (pleasant) or negative (unpleasant) and to some extent also as arousing or quieting.

Positive affect is generally short-lasting but is energizing and associated with creativity and divergent thinking. Positive affect is also closely associated with vitality and happiness. In contrast, negative affect often depletes a person's energy, is associated with avoidance tendencies, and limits the person's problem-solving potential. Negative affect can easily turn into a chronic and self-sustaining state.

In contrast, emotion, as we defined it earlier, is a multidimensional construct that also includes, aside from the affective experience, motivational tendencies and contextual and cultural factors. This then results in a complex experience that can be regulated to some extent through intra- and interpersonal processes.

Because emotional episodes are reactions to something, the cognitive appraisal involved in the transaction between person and object is a defining element. An important feature of affect for the purpose of our discussion is that there are individual differences in the way people deal with emotional information. Similar to cognitive schemas that give rise to specific maladaptive thoughts by overestimating unlikely but dangerous outcomes, some approaches to emotional information (affective styles) can also be maladaptive if they lead to excessive distress or behavioral problems (i.e., if the person experiences more distress or interference than most other people would experience in a similar situation).

CORE AFFECT

Despite the complexity of emotions, modern emotion theorists tend to agree that any affect (i.e., any subjective experience of an emotional state) includes two basic dimensions: activation versus deactivation (also referred to as the dimension of "arousal") and pleasantness versus unpleasantness (also referred to as the dimension of "valence"). This model has become known as the *affective circumplex model* (Posner, Russell, & Peterson, 2005; Russell, 1980; Colibazzi et al., 2010). The dimensions in this model have also been referred to as *core affect* (e.g., Russell, 2003; Russell & Barrett, 1999) because they describe the simplest and most elementary feelings that serve as building blocks for any other, more complex emotional experiences.

This model describes any subjective emotional experience by its valence and arousal. The valence dimension refers to the hedonic tone of the subjective experience of the emotion, whereas arousal determines the degree of activation, which is associated with physiological alertness and responsiveness. Some examples of adjectives that describe emotional experiences are provided in Figure 1.1. (A more recent and more elaborate version of this model is discussed in Yik, Russell, & Steiger, 2011.) For example, *excited* is a pleasant and activated emotional state, whereas *relaxed* is a pleasant and deactivated emotional state. In contrast, *being bored* is an unpleasant and deactivated state, whereas being *nervous* is an unpleasant and activated state.

The valence–arousal circumplex is one of the most widely empirically supported dimensional models of affect (see Russell & Barrett, 1999, for a review). And yet, despite its parsimony, utility, and robustness, the model may not fully account for all individual differences in the experience and representations of affect (Feldman, 1995a, 1995b; Remington, Fabrigar, & Visser, 2000; Terracciano, McCrae, Hagemann, & Costa, 2003; Watson, Wiese, Vaidya, & Tellegen, 1999). Nevertheless, it provides a useful model to simplify and describe the complexity of emotional experiences.

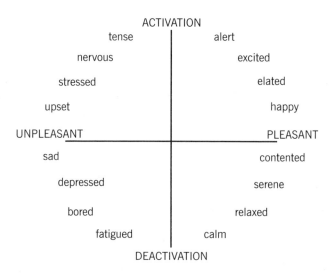

FIGURE 1.1. Any emotional experience is a point in this two-dimensional space. The horizontal axis represents the valence dimension (pleasant–unpleasant), whereas the vertical axis represents the arousal dimension of an emotion. Examples of adjectives that describe emotions are added. From Colibazzi et al. (2010). Copyright 2010 by the American Psychological Association. Reprinted by permission.

In Practice: Distinguishing Arousal from Pleasantness

Emotions are complex, and the question "How are you feeling?" is difficult to answer. The answers "good" and "bad" are unspecific and undifferentiated, but they provide a rough categorization of the experience on the valence dimension. However, clearly more information is required. The first step when targeting emotional distress is to become aware of the many shades of the emotional experience.

Adding the dimension of arousal/activation provides meaningful additional information. For example, depression is a state of unpleasant deactivation; being relaxed is a state of pleasant deactivation; fear is a state of unpleasant activation; and being excited is a state of pleasant activation. Any emotional experience corresponds to a point on this *affect grid* (see Figure 1.2).

In order for patients to gain a more fine-grained awareness of their emotions, they may be asked to monitor their arousal and pleasantness. For example, for a period of time (e.g., 2 weeks), a patient may be asked to place some dots in the grid in Figure 1.2 to indicate how he or she is feeling at a given moment, using the two basic dimensions of arousal/activation and pleasantness.

The therapist might also ask the patient to record his or her emotions using these dimensions at the same times every day (e.g., 8:00 A.M., 2:00 P.M., and 5:00 P.M.). This assessment time could be tied to a particular routine (e.g., right before the patient leaves for work, after lunch, after coming home, etc.). Initially, the patient should not wait for a significant event to arise (e.g., an argument with spouse) but develop a regular assessment schedule of monitoring her or his emotional state.

The goal is to get a sense of one's emotional life throughout a normal day. The resulting picture becomes a reflection of the person's emotional life during a normal day (assuming that there are no unusual events happening during this time). This exercise can clarify whether there is a specific pattern to the patient's emotional experiences. If the patient's emotional life is relatively flat (i.e., without many highs and lows and with moderate activation), the dots will cluster around the zero point (i.e., where the two dimensions intersect). Regular changes in mood will result in dots clustered in a certain quadrant; otherwise, they will be distributed across the grid. This exercise can raise awareness of the patient's emotional experience and can identify patterns in subtle mood swings throughout the day that the person might not be aware of.

Again, a specific pattern can provide information that is usually difficult to identify. For example, a happy person might place many dots located on the right (pleasant) side of the grid, whereas depressed and anxious people might place many dots to the left (unpleasant).

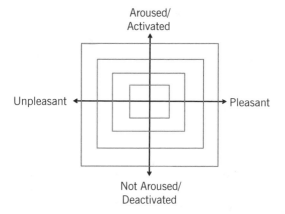

Instructions: Place a mark in this grid to indicate how pleasant (or unpleasant) and how aroused/activated an emotional experience made then feel. You can use the same grid for all of the emotional experiences you have had within a certain time period.

FIGURE 1.2. An affect grid that shows the dimensions of arousal/activation and nonarousal/deactivation. From *Emotion in Therapy: From Science to Practice* by Stefan G. Hofmann. Copyright © 2016 by The Guilford Press. Permission to photocopy this figure is granted to purchasers of this book for personal use or use with individual clients (see copyright page for details). Purchasers can download an enlarged version of this figure (see the box at the end of the table of contents).

POSITIVE VERSUS NEGATIVE AFFECT

Positive and negative affect are mutually inhibitory. The *broaden-and-build model* (e.g., Fredrickson, 2000) assumes that positive affect loosens the influence of negative affect on the person and at the same time broadens the behavioral repertoire by enhancing physical, social, and intellectual resources. In addition, positive affect has a direct inhibitory effect on emotion disorders. In essence, happiness and joy directly counter emotional disorders such as depression, anxiety, and anger control problems.

However, the inhibitory influence of positive affect is easily overshadowed by negative affect if the negative affect cannot be regulated adaptively. The dysregulation of negative affect is the direct cause of emotional disorder. A positive feedback loop is established from the disorder to the dysregulation, negative affect, and affective style, leading to a chronic condition that becomes difficult to change. A more in-depth discussion of emotional disorders is provided in Chapter 2.

FUNCTION OF EMOTIONS

As noted by Darwin, emotions have an adaptive communicative function, both within and between species. Emotions are closely linked to the social system of the organism, because many emotional experiences and expressions serve important roles in social communication. In fact, one could argue that without social connections, emotions such as shame, jealousy, and embarrassment would not exist. Other emotions can arise outside of the social relationship with peers. For example, one can experience anger toward members of another species (e.g., a dog) nonliving objects, (e.g., a car that doesn't start), or oneself, or sadness because of a loss of a valued object. In many cases, of course, emotions are not uniquely linked to any particular context.

In many (but not all) such cases, anger has a communicative function (as in the case of anger toward another person or toward a dog). Anger toward the car is either noncommunicative or a misguided form of communication (because the car cannot be a recipient in the communication). Mayr (1974) distinguished between behaviors directed toward the living and the nonliving worlds (communicative vs. noncommunicative behaviors). Within the communicative category, Mayr further distinguished between behaviors that are directed toward members of one's own species (intraspecific behaviors) and behaviors that are directed toward members of other species (interspecific behaviors). Different emotional problems map onto different behaviors of Mayr's classification system. For example, in the case of anxiety disorders, the fears of heights, snakes, and social situations correspond to noncommunicative, interspecific communicative, and intraspecific communicative behaviors, respectively. The communicative function of emotions has also been referred to as *instrumental* if they serve a particular purpose to achieve a certain aim (e.g., Greenberg, 2011; Greenberg & Paivio, 1997). For example, people may show sadness to elicit empathy from others, or they may show anger in order to intimidate others.

As such, emotions may be viewed as evolved mechanisms with an adaptive function and at times a communicative value. In general, evolved psychological mechanisms are believed to be sets of processes that have developed into their current form as a result of solving specific adaptive problems for our ancestors (Buss, 1999).

An adaptive solution is one that increases the inclusive fitness of the individual, meaning that his or her genes have an increased chance of being represented in subsequent generations (Hamilton, 1964). For example, fear protects oneself, avoids harm, and promotes survival; shame leads to remorse and a decreased likelihood that the shameful behavior is shown in the future (Plutchik, 1980).

Emotions and their communicative role thus appear to occupy important functions to promote survival of the genes and species. In humans, listening and speaking are accompanied and regulated by expressions of emotion, such as nods, eye contact, smiles, postural shifts, vocalizations, and so forth (e.g., Plutchik, 2000). These communicative signals through emotional expressions can happen on a conscious or an unconscious level. We can read "between the lines" and are confused about receiving "mixed messages" when the spoken words are inconsistent with the emotional expressions.

Some emotion theorists assume that positive and negative affect are bipolar opposites (Russell & Carroll, 1999), whereas others (e.g., Fredrickson, 2000) believe that positive and negative affect can coexist and serve different functions. Clinically, it is evident that somebody who does not experience negative affect does not necessarily experience positive affect. Similarly, the lack of a positive affect does not imply the presence of negative affect. Moreover, one might experience both negative and positive affect at the same time—joy and fear (such as during a roller coaster ride), ecstasy and terror (while parachute jumping), happiness and sadness (when thinking of a loved one who passed away some time ago).

Whereas emotions with negatively valenced (unpleasant) affect, such as fear, anger, and sadness, are assumed to be associated with a limited behavioral repertoire in a given situation (e.g., fear is more likely associated with escape behaviors, whereas anger is more likely associated with aggressive behaviors), emotions with pleasant affect, such as joy, interest, and contentment, are assumed to broaden the behavioral repertoire. For example, fear is typically an emotion that is associated with escape or avoidance from a particular object or situation, whereas anger is typically associated with aggression and approach. The behavioral repertoires of both emotions include a relatively limited set of specific behavioral tendencies focused on specific objects or situations (e.g., running away from a specific predator or running toward a particular enemy). In contrast, positive emotions, such as joy, interest, and contentment, typically include a multitude of nonspecific behavioral and approach-related tendencies associated with a number of sensorial experiences. For example, the joy one experiences after reaching the peak of a mountain includes the sounds, smells, and sights of the surroundings, the smiles of one's companions, and so forth.

NATURE VERSUS NURTURE

The nature-versus-nurture distinction is an important issue in emotion research. Some contemporary authors reject the notion that there are basic, biologically hardwired emotions (e.g., Barrett, Mesquita, Ochsner, & Gross, 2007). Instead, an emotional experience is conceptualized as a transient, context-dependent phenomenon that results from an affective state with some degree of arousal that is experienced as either pleasurable or unpleasant (referred to earlier as *core affect*; e.g., Barrett et al., 2007; Russell, 2003) and the association between this state and the person's knowledge about the emotional experience. Therefore, *core affect* is not the same as an emotion; core affect is one aspect of the more complex construct called emotion, as defined earlier. Contextual and cultural factors are important determinants in the experience of an emotion. For example, if a person is confronted with a rattlesnake while hiking, he or she will experience unpleasant affect, which may be categorized and labeled as *fear*, depending on his or her knowledge about poisonous snakes. Of course, this model stands in contrast to the biological and Darwinian conceptualization of emotions and the view that a sight of a snake can trigger an innate fear response (e.g., Poulton & Menzies, 2002). The relative contributions of biology (and nature) versus culture (and nurture) is an issue of ongoing debate in the contemporary emotion literature. For the purpose of our discussion, emotion is considered, dy defined, as a multidimensional and biologically based construct that is shaped by contextual and cultural factors and that can be regulated to some extent by intrapersonal and interpersonal processes. Thus, this conceptualization acknowledges both nature and nurture, with a particular focus on the social and cognitive factors that modulate the experience and expression of emotions.

METAEXPERIENCE OF EMOTIONS

People are not only able to feel emotions, such as fear, anger, sadness, or happiness, but they are also able to feel emotions about the emotions. This metaexperience is a basic focus of a psychodynamically oriented treatment that has become known as emotion-focused therapy (EFT; Greenberg, 2011). Specifically, EFT distinguishes between *primary emotions* and *secondary emotions* and also classifies certain emotions as *instrumental emotions*. All of these forms of emotions can be *adaptive* (i.e., generally acceptable emotions that do not cause long-lasting problems) or *maladaptive* (i.e., emotions that lead to persistent psychological or interpersonal problems). *Instrumental emotions* are emotions (or, more accurately, behaviors associated with emotions) that serve a particular function. For example, a child might cry in order to manipulate others to comfort him or her, thus allowing the child to escape punishment. *Primary emotions* are the most fundamental responses to a certain event or situation. Primary adaptive emotions prepare the individual for adaptive response and usually subside when the situation changes or when the basic needs are met. In contrast, primary maladaptive emotions are often assumed to be connected to earlier traumatic experiences and usually do not subside quickly. *Secondary emotions* are responses to primary emotions or to cognitions rather than to the eliciting situation or event. For example, a breakup with a boyfriend may lead to sadness (the primary emotion), and the grieving girlfriend might also experience anger about her sadness (the secondary emotion). Secondary emotions can serve a defensive function (e.g., being angry may protect against experiencing more vulnerable sadness). In addition, secondary emotions may be activated in response to thoughts, such as when people feel anxious in response to worries or ashamed in response to violent fantasies.

Such perceptions and appraisals of emotional experiences have been described as *metaexperiences of emotions* (Mayer & Gaschke, 1988). In other words, one might perceive an emotion as problematic or aversive, which in turn can influence the way the person regulates his or her emotional states. Perceiving an emotion as being problematic can also cause confusion about one's emotional state and lead one to use avoidance strategies to manage the confusing emotional experience.

An illustrative example might be a divorced husband (Charlie) who feels relief at being out of the marriage but also a great deal of anger about his love for his estranged wife. Charlie and his wife divorced because both realized that the relationship was broken beyond repair after too many hurtful fights and extramarital affairs. Although it is clear that there is no more future for them as a couple, Charlie still loves his ex-wife. At the same time, he wants to move on and date other women again. But loving his ex-wife makes it hard to start anew. As a result, Charlie feels anger at his love for his ex-wife—an emotion (anger) about another (incongruent) emotion (love)—which can lead to a great deal of emotional confusion that can hold him back from living a happy life with another person.

More complex cases may include the sadness that arises when experiencing love toward another person or a feeling of both fear and guilt experienced by the rape victim when remembering the horror of the rape. Such mixed emotional experiences often leave a person in a state of confusion.

In Practice: Raising Awareness of Metaexperiences

A phenomenon related to metaemotion is metacognition: thoughts about thoughts. For example, people who worry excessively about the future or about minor matters might not only experience elevated and chromic anxiety but might also hold certain beliefs about their worries (e.g., "worrying will keep me safe"). Other beliefs might even take on the form of worries about worries ("I will lose my mind if I worry too much"). In therapy, monitoring a client's emotions about emotions (metaemotions) and thoughts about thoughts can identify certain patterns that might be responsible for the maintenance of his or her problem.

Figure 1.3 is a simple tool that clients can use to monitor the relationship between the chain of specific thoughts and feelings on two levels to identify

Instructions: Describe the initial situation (e.g., "bungee jumping"), the thought that comes to mind (e.g., "I will get hurt"), and the feeling associated with this thought (e.g., "fear"). Next, examine the second-level thought that comes to mind when you have this feeling. For example, you might think "I am a wimp" because you feel fear. Next, examine the feeling associated with this thought (e.g., "embarrassment").

Situation (e.g., bungee jumping)	Thought 1 about Situation (e.g., "I will get hurt.")	Feeling 1 about Thought 1 (e.g., fear)	Thought 2 about Feeling 1 (e.g., "I am such a wimp.")	Feeling 2 about Thought 2 (e.g., embarrassment)

FIGURE 1.3. Monitoring first- and second-level thoughts and emotions.

overarching schemas. This tool can be used in session and as a homework monitoring sheet for patients. When using this sheet, the client is asked to first report her or his thought (e.g., "I will get hurt") about a particular situation (e.g., bungee jumping), her or his feeling about this initial thought (e.g., fear), the second-level thought about this feeling (e.g., "I am such a wimp"), and the second level feeling about this second-level thought (e.g., "I am embarrassed").

Summary of Clinically Relevant Points

- An emotion is (1) a multidimensional experience that is (2) characterized by different levels of arousal and degrees of pleasure–displeasure; (3) associated with subjective experiences, somatic sensations, and motivational tendencies; and (4) colored by contextual and cultural factors; and that (5) can be regulated to some degree through intra- and interpersonal processes.

- The affective circumplex model provides a framework to classify emotional experiences based on the two core affect dimensions: activation–deactivation and pleasantness–unpleasantness.

- In order to enhance emotional awareness, patients may be instructed to monitor their emotional states using an affect grid at particular times during the day and after significant events.

- Once patients become more aware of the nature of their emotions, they may be asked to label an emotional experience using common emotional adjectives. Pure emotions rarely exist. Much more typical are blends of different emotions.

- Some emotions have an important communicative function by providing cues about an internal state. People differ in their ability or willingness to signal and read emotions in other people.

- In order to gain further clarity about their emotional states, patients may be instructed to explore not only their thoughts and feelings about specific events or triggers but also their thoughts and feelings about their initial/primary feelings. Behaviors and physiological symptoms can precede and cause emotions, and emotions can also precede and cause behaviors and physiological symptoms.

CHAPTER TWO

◆

Individual Differences

People differ in many ways. Some are tall; others are short. Some are heavily built and struggle with their weight, whereas others are thin and are able to maintain a similar weight throughout their adult lives. People also differ in their intelligence, temperaments, and personalities. Are some of these traits linked to emotions? Do people differ in their emotional responses to the same situation? If so, why? Are there specific strategies people use to cope with their emotions? Are some of these strategies linked to emotional disorders?

This chapter attempts to provide some answers to these complicated questions. I discuss the different biological and psychological factors that contribute to these individual differences. Some factors are easier to assess than others. (A number of commonly used and brief self-report instruments to assess some of these difference variables are listed in Appendix I at the end of the book.) I integrate the various factors into a diathesis–stress model of emotional disorders at the end of this chapter.

LEVELS OF INDIVIDUAL DIFFERENCES

As defined in Chapter 1, an emotion is a multidimensional experience that is characterized by different levels of arousal and degrees of pleasure–displeasure (some people experience greater arousal and pleasure to the same stimuli than others do), that is associated with subjective experiences (some people will respond with a qualitatively different type of affect to the same situation than others), somatic sensations, and motivational tendencies (different individuals will have different motives), and that is colored by contextual and cultural factors (different cultures shape affective experiences in particular ways). As already noted, an emotion can be regulated to some degree through intra- and interpersonal processes.

Traditionally, emotion researchers have primarily focused on general characteristics of emotions that are common to all people and that even cut across different species. Other researchers have examined individual differences in the experience of emotions (Feldman, 1995a, 1995b; Remington et al., 2000; Terracciano et al., 2003; Watson et al., 1999; Winter & Kuiper, 1997).

Acknowledging and understanding these differences are essential in translating findings from the emotion research literature into clinical practice. In this chapter, I review the role of the environment and the person's diathesis in the development and maintenance of emotional disorders. A central element of the model that I present here is the person's affective style, which can lead to a predominance of negative affect and a deficiency of positive affect, and the maladaptive strategies for coping with negative affect that eventually lead to emotional disorders.

CULTURAL BACKGROUND

It is important to consider the person's individual background in this discussion. Sexual orientation, culture, socioeconomic and education status, trauma history, physical disabilities, and so forth are all important factors that determine the person's individual background. It is impossible to provide a balanced and in-depth discussion of all of these important factors within the boundaries of this volume.

Instead, I briefly focus on only one of these background factors: the influence of culture on emotions.

Emotional well-being is strongly influenced by cultural factors (Hofstede, 1984). Culture is an important context that modulates individual differences in emotional experiences. An important aspect on which cultures differ is individualism and collectivism. Collectivism describes the relationship between members of social organizations that emphasizes the interdependence of their members. In collectivistic cultures, harmony within the group is the highest priority, and individual gain is considered to be less important than improvement of the broader social group. In contrast, in individualistic societies, individual achievements and success receive the greatest reward and social admiration. It has been shown that social contacts serve different purposes in individualistic versus collectivistic cultures (Lucas, Diener, & Grob, 2000). In individualistic cultures, individual feelings and thoughts more directly determine behavior. In collectivistic cultures, social norms and role expectations have a considerable impact on behavior. Therefore, the subjective sense of well-being and happiness is also more dependent on social contact in collectivistic than in individualistic societies. Self-esteem was more highly correlated with life satisfaction in individualistic than in collectivist cultures (Diener & Diener, 1995).

There are also cultural differences in the association between congruence (i.e., acting consistently across situations and in accord with oneself) and life satisfaction. In South Korea, for example, congruence is much less important than in the United States. Moreover, people in collectivist cultures more often rely on social norms to decide whether they should be satisfied and consider the social appraisals of family and friends in evaluating their lives (Suh, Diener, Oishi, & Triandis, 1998). People in collectivist cultures, as compared with individualistic societies, are more likely to remain in marriages and jobs that they are unhappy in, possibly because they attempt to conform to social norms and perhaps because people in troubled marriages and jobs are more likely to get support from others (Diener, 2000). People differ in their cultural backgrounds and upbringing, especially those who live in a multicultural society such as the United States. Despite the differences in cultures (as well as many other factors), there are a number of common influences that determine the individual differences in emotional experiences. These include psychological and biological vulnerabilities, which I subsume under the more general term *diathesis*.

DIATHESIS

Temperament

A general diathesis to individual differences in emotion regulation is *temperament*, which refers to a person's general character or traits. The most widely studied temperament is shyness. Longitudinal studies in children have shown that a person's response to novel situations or social stress is remarkably consistent throughout the years, starting in infancy and continuing well into adulthood (for a review, see Kagan & Snidman, 2004). Moreover, adults who were classified as being shy in the second year of life showed greater amygdala activation (the brain structure involved in fear) to novel versus familiar faces as compared with those previously categorized as nonshy (Schwartz, Wright, Shin, Kagan, & Rauch, 2003).

The results show that some temperamental aspects are greatly determined by genetic factors and remarkably consistent throughout one's lifetime. These data are also consistent with the notion that people who are not overly shy are better able to modulate their hedonic tone in a more positive direction more effectively than shy people.

Emotional Granularity

Individual differences already exist on the affect level. In order to account for individual differences in the valence–arousal circumplex model, Feldman Barrett (Barrett, 2004; Feldman, 1995a, 1995b) introduced the *emotional granularity* concept. Emotional granularity refers to the ability to distinguish among emotional states and is a function of how information about valence and arousal is incorporated into representations of emotions (Barrett, 2004). Individuals high in granularity represent their emotional states with high specificity (i.e., the person is able to distinguish between similar emotional states, such as anger and annoyance), whereas individuals low in granularity represent their emotional states in more global terms (i.e., all negatively valenced emotional states are represented as "feeling bad").

Emotional granularity can be arousal-focused, valence-focused, or both. *Arousal focus* refers to the amount of information about arousal or intensity (i.e., activation and deactivation) that is contained in representations of an emotion, whereas *valence focus* refers to the degree to which information about the valence (i.e., unpleasantness and pleasantness) is contained in representations of emotions. Individuals high in both arousal and valence focus incorporate information about both the pleasantness and activation of their experience in their verbal reports of emotion. Such individuals are better able to distinguish among emotional states than others.

Although emotional granularity is highly relevant for mental disorders, little research exists on it in clinical populations. Studies have found that patients with schizophrenia (Kring, Barrett, & Gard, 2003) and borderline personality disorder (Suvak et al., 2001) weighted valence more and arousal less than normal people in their mental representations of affect, pointing to a greater degree of disorganization in the representations of emotions in the clinical groups.

Alexithymia

The concept *alexithymia* grew out of the psychodynamic and psychosomatic literature and has been defined as the difficulty in identifying and describing subjective feelings; difficulty distinguishing between feelings and the bodily sensations of emotional arousal; constricted imaginal capacities, as evidenced by a paucity of fantasies; and an externally oriented cognitive style (Nemiah, Freyberger, & Sifneos, 1976). More recently, it has been defined as deficits in the cognitive processing and regulation of emotions (Taylor, Bagby, & Parker, 1997).

People with high degrees of alexithymia are assumed to be limited in their ability to reflect on and regulate their emotions and to verbally communicate emotional distress to other people, thereby failing to enlist others as sources of aid or comfort. They have difficulties identifying and describing emotions, they minimize emotional experiences, and they tend to focus their attention externally. Moreover, they are assumed to have constricted imaginal capacities that limit the extent to which they can modulate emotions by fantasy, dreams, interests, and play.

Alexithymia appears to be associated with maladaptive styles of emotion regulation, such as bingeing on food or developing a headache, and negatively with adaptive behaviors, such as thinking about and trying to understand distressing feelings or talking to a caring person (Taylor et al., 1997). Many of the cognitive skills required to effectively monitor and self-regulate emotions are encompassed in the construct of emotional intelligence.

Emotional Clarity

The counterpart to alexithymia is emotional clarity, which refers to the awareness and understanding of one's own emotions and emotional experiences, as well as the ability to properly label them (Gohm & Clore, 2000). High levels of emotional clarity have been linked to adaptive coping and positive well-being (Gohm & Clore, 2000), whereas low emotional clarity predicts maladaptive interpersonal responses to stress and depressive symptoms in youth (Flynn & Rudolph, 2010).

It has further been shown that encouraging patients to label their emotions has beneficial treatment effects. This has been nicely demonstrated in a study by Kircanski, Lieberman, and Craske (2012). The authors repeatedly exposed patients to a live spider. Some patients were asked to label their emotions, others were asked to reappraise the situation, a third group was instructed to distract themselves, and a fourth group received no specific instructions during the brief exposure treatment. One week later, all patients were retested in a different context and exposed to a different spider. The affect-labeling group exhibited a greater reduction in skin conductance response relative to the other groups and had a marginally greater tendency to approach the spider than the distraction group. Moreover, the more often patients used anxiety and fear words during the exposure, the greater the reductions in fear responding was.

However, as already discussed in Chapter 1, emotions, especially in clinical practice, rarely come in pure forms, and they tend to change over time. For example, our response to the death of a relative might turn from overwhelming sadness and loneliness to guilt caused by anger and resentment at being left behind. Emotions change both in intensity and quality (e.g., sadness slowly becomes less intense and is replaced by other emotions), and some emotions can cause other emotions (e.g., guilt at feeling anger toward the deceased person or positive affect, such as relief). Some people who experience, for example, relief over the death of a loved one might experience psychological distress because of that emotion (which could result in complicated grief in some cases).

In brief, and as noted in Chapter 1, emotions are "messy" because emotional experiences often consist of blends of a variety of different, and sometimes contradictory, emotions (e.g., feeling happy, sad, and proud when a child moves out of the family house to start college). Similar to a painting, an emotional experience consists of many different colors and shades of colors of different intensities. Sometimes, a painting consists of similar colors that differ in intensities; at other times, it consists of opposing colors. So, too, an affective experience can consist of similarly valenced emotions that differ in arousal; at other times, the experience may comprise emotions with seemingly contradictory valences (i.e., sometimes an emotional experience can include both pleasant and unpleasant affect).

In Practice: Clarifying Emotions

In order to gain a better understanding about the type of emotions a patient experiences, it can be useful to instruct the client to label them by using a pie chart. The whole pie reflects the entirety of the emotional experience; the various slices are components that make up the experience at any given time.

Imagine the emotional experience of a wife whose loving husband, Bob, passed away after a 20-year marriage. As with any marriage, some aspects were good, others not so good. Sadness and loneliness are clearly the most socially acceptable emotions associated with his death. But even a loving wife might have positive feelings associated with her new freedom. Although she might have loved Bob, some of his behaviors might have had some negative consequences on her life. She always wanted to further pursue her hobby as a painter, but Bob was not supportive of it. Now she has the opportunity to paint and become an artist. At the same time, she is also a devout Catholic who is prepared to undergo a prolonged grieving period for her husband. Her excitement about the prospect of pursuing her passion might, in turn, lead to feelings of guilt and shame or even depression and self-hate. The pie chart labeling her feelings (see Figure 2.1) can clarify her conflictual feelings about Bob's death.

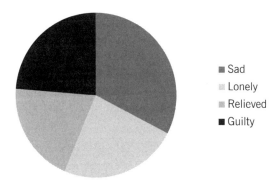

FIGURE 2.1. Patient's feelings about Bob's death.

Emotional Intelligence

The term *emotional intelligence* includes the ability to identify and label one's own and other people's emotional states, the ability to express emotions accurately and make empathic responses to other people, and the ability to reflect upon emotions and use them in adaptive ways. More generally speaking, emotional intelligence includes skills from the following three categories of adaptive abilities: (1) appraisal and expression of emotions, (2) regulation of emotions, and (3) utilization of emotions in solving problems (Mayer & Salovey, 1997; Salovey & Mayer, 1990). In other words, a person with high emotional intelligence is able to quickly and accurately assess and interpret an emotion, can regulate his or her own emotion effectively, and can use emotions as a way to solve problems. The ability to appraise and express an emotion involves the verbal and nonverbal perception of emotions and empathy, and the utilization of emotions requires the ability to flexibly plan, think creatively, and redirect attention and motivation (Salovey & Mayer, 1990).

In a more recent reformulation of the definition of emotional intelligence, a greater emphasis is placed on the cognitive components of emotional intelligence, which provide the potential for intellectual and emotional growth (Mayer & Salovey, 1997). This revised conceptualization of emotional intelligence distinguishes four components or branches: (1) perception; (2) appraisal and expression of emotion; (3) emotional facilitation of thinking, understanding, analyzing, and employing emotional knowledge; and (4) reflective regulation of emotions to further emotional and intellectual growth. Each branch is associated with specific levels of skills, which individuals master in sequential order. Accordingly, the components perception, appraisal, and expression of emotion are viewed as the most basic, whereas the ability to reflectively regulate emotions is considered to be the most complex process.

The notion that emotional intelligence requires a number of specific cognitive, social, and communication skills for understanding and expressing emotions is shared by other researchers (Cooper & Sawaf, 1997; Goleman, 1995). Some of these skills include emotional literacy, emotional fitness, emotional depth, and "emotional alchemy" (Cooper & Sawaf, 1997). Emotional literacy includes knowledge of one's own emotions and how they function; emotional fitness includes emotional hardiness and flexibility; emotional depth involves emotional intensity and potential for growth; and "emotional alchemy" includes the ability to use emotion to spark creativity.

Distress Tolerance

The degree to which a person can tolerate negative affect is key to understanding individual differences in emotions. Distress tolerance is the ability to experience unpleasant internal states without being overwhelmed or rendered unable to function. This ability is associated with various forms of psychopathology (Leyro, Zvolensky, & Bernstein, 2010). People who are unable to tolerate distress are more likely to employ emotional avoidance and suppression strategies to regulate negative affect. In contrast, individuals with high distress tolerance are more willing to experience a high level of negative affect without employing any avoidance strategies. Mindfulness exercises, which encourage the person to experience the here and now in an open, curious, and nonjudgmental manner, seem to be effective at regulating distress because they strengthen a person's distress tolerance of negative affect (Bullis, Boe, Asnaani, Hofmann, 2014; Feldman, Dunn, Stemke, Bell, & Greeson, 2014). These exercises are discussed in more detail in Chapter 7 along with simple relaxation practices that can be effective at lowering emotional arousal.

AFFECTIVE STYLES

The term *affective style* refers to the interindividual difference in the habitual use of strategies to cope with emotional information. Different affective styles (or coping strategies) can be identified.

Problem-Focused versus Emotion-Focused Coping

Coping strategies can be generally classified as either problem-focused or emotion-focused. Problem-focused coping seems to be more appropriate for controllable stress (such as the stress that comes from accepting too many invitations to write academic papers), whereas emotion-focused coping appears to be more appropriate for stress that is perceived as uncontrollable (such as the stress that comes from exposure to an assault or a natural disaster; Compas, Malcarne, & Fondacaro, 1988; Folkman & Moskowitz, 2004; Lazarus & Folkman, 1984; Vitaliano, DeWolfe, Mairuro, Russo, & Katon, 1990).

A simple illustration of problem-focused versus emotion-focused coping is the case of Mary and Scott. Mary has been married to Scott for 10 years. They have a generally good relationship, but Scott is not overly helpful around the house. This makes Mary occasionally very upset. In addition, Scott is bothered by Mary's snoring, which often keeps him up at night. As a result, he has developed a great degree of anger toward her. Simple examples of problem-focused and emotion-focused coping strategies are listed in Figure 2.2.

Styles of Emotion-Focused Coping

Given the same situation, some affective styles are more likely to lead to positive affect, whereas others are more likely to lead to negative affect. Affective styles determine people's general approaches toward dealing with the emotional world, similar to some cognitive schemas that determine the likelihood estimates of catastrophic outcomes. Davidson and Begley (2012) recently proposed the existence of six emotional style dimensions or continua and assume that the combination of a person's positions on all the dimensions results in the overall emotional style. The first style is the *resiliency style*. This style refers to how quickly or slowly a person recovers from adversity. Some people take a long time to recover, whereas others are able to

Problem	Problem-focused coping: Directed toward reducing or eliminating the problem	Emotion-focused coping: Directed toward changing one's emotional response to the problem
Mary is bothered by Scott's messiness.	Come up with schedule and cleaning assignments for Scott.	Discuss her feelings with Scott to calm her down.
	Get cleaning lady to tidy up regularly.	Talk to friend or counselor about her feelings.
Scott is angry about Mary's snoring.	Get Mary to see a doctor to treat her snoring problem.	Discuss his feelings with Mary to reduce his anger.
	Sleep in a different room or use earplugs.	Talk to friend or counselor about his anger.

FIGURE 2.2. Examples of problem-focused versus emotion-focused coping strategies.

recover very quickly. The second style is the *outlook style*. It refers to how long positive affect persists and is associated with the propensity to view the world in either a positive or a negative light. The third style is the *social intuition style*. It refers to how accurately a person is able to decode others' nonverbal signals of emotion. The fourth style is the *self-awareness style*. This style refers to the accuracy with which a person decodes the internal bodily cues of emotions, such as heart rate and muscle tension. Some people are acutely aware of their own internal states, whereas others are not. The fifth dimension is the *context style*, which refers to sensitivity to context. Some people are better, others worse at modulating their emotional responses in context-appropriate ways. Finally, the sixth dimension is the *attention style*, reflecting the fact that some people are more focused at particular tasks and are better able to resist emotional stimuli that would pull their attention away from the task at hand than are others. These emotional styles are implicit in many of the constructs and themes that are covered in this book.

When limiting the use of the term *style* to emotion regulation (rather than to emotion in general), the literature consistently identifies suppression and other strategies aimed at concealing and avoiding emotions after they arise (*concealing* style). Other people are more able to access and use emotional information in adaptive ways toward problem solving and are better able to modulate emotional experience and expression according to contextual demands (Mennin, Heimberg, Turk, & Fresco, 2005; Hofmann, Sawyer, Fang, & Asnaani, 2012). These individuals possess the tools to readjust or balance emotions as needed to successfully navigate the rewards and punishments of everyday life (*adjusting* style). Finally, a third style reflects comfort and nondefensiveness in response to arousing emotional experiences as they exist in the present moment. This style, which includes mindfulness and acceptance strategies, allows tolerating strong emotions (*tolerating* style; see Hofmann et al., 2012).

Emotional Flexibility

Emotional flexibility is the ability to adjust one's emotion regulation strategies to the demands of a given situation in order to effectively meet or cope with those demands (Aldao, 2013; Bonanno & Burton, 2013; Bonnano, Papa, O'Neil, Westphal, & Coifman, 2004; Cheng, 2001; Consedine, Magai, & Bonanno, 2002; Kashdan & Rottenberg, 2010; Sheppes et al., 2014). People with this ability flexibly adjust to a challenge by either suppressing or enhancing their emotional experience (e.g., suppressing the intensity of the affect arousal or enhancing the affect valence associated with an emotion). Emotional flexibility is closely associated with the more general term *psychological flexibility,* which is the ability to adapt to a variety of different situational demands by shifting one's mind-set or behaviors (Kashdan & Rottenberg, 2010). Similarly, it has been assumed that it is coping flexibility, rather than the use of any specific coping strategy per se, that best predicts successful adaption to challenging situations.

It has been shown that people differ in their tendency to use specific coping strategies for various real-life stressful events, over a 3-month time period, and in laboratory settings (Cheng, 2001). Approximately 30% of participants showed a considerable degree of variability in their designation of stressors as desirable and in the extent to which they perceive the stressors as controllable and also showed variability in their deployment of problem-focused or emotion-focused coping strategies. These individuals showed better daily adjustment and less anxiety and depression over the course of a 1-week period as compared with people who showed a rigid adherence to a particular kind of coping strategy, regardless of whether this strategy was emotion-focused or problem-focused (Cheng, 2003). Similarly, it has been shown that emotional flexibility is associated with reduced levels of subjective distress in individuals entering college (Bonanno et al., 2004).

DYSREGULATION OF NEGATIVE AFFECT: RUMINATION, BROODING, AND WORRYING

Rumination, brooding, and worrying are cognitive processes that are implicated in maladaptive attempts to cope with stress. All three activities are characterized by repetitive processes that focus on symptoms, causes, and consequences of one's distress (Nolen-Hoeksema, Wisco, & Lyubomirsky, 2008). Rumination is a multifactorial construct consisting of brooding and reflection. Brooding is the cognitive activity of focusing on symptoms of distress, whereas reflection emphasizes active efforts to gain insights into one's problems (Treynor, Gonzalez, & Nolen-Hoeksema, 2003). Both aspects of rumination are typically correlated with depression in cross-sectional analyses, with brooding showing stronger associations (Nolen-Hoeksema et al., 2008; Treynor et al., 2003).

Whereas rumination is an attempt to cope with past events, worrying is a maladaptive cognitive activity that focuses on future events. Worrying and rumination primarily involve verbal activity and, to a lesser extent, imagery. Imagery and verbal processes have different effects on the psychophysiological response to emotional material. For example, verbalizing a fearful situation typically induces less cardiovascular response than visually imagining the same situation, possibly because verbalizations are used as a strategy for abstraction and disengagement. This suggests that the verbal activity during worrying is less closely connected to the affective, physiological, and behavioral systems than images are and, therefore, verbalizing might be a poor vehicle for processing emotional information (Borkovec, Ray, & Stöber, 1998). Worrying has even been conceptualized as a cognitive avoidance strategy. For example, worries about being late to work could be linked to a fear of losing one's job or even more catastrophic scenarios, such as continuous unemployment, bankruptcy, divorce, homelessness, and so forth. Thus worrying about minor matters may be a way to avoid the worst-case scenario. Such worst-case scenarios can best be described and processed by using imagery.

Worrying seems further associated with intolerance of uncertainty, a cognitive vulnerability factor and dispositional variable for chronic anxiety (Ladouceur, Gosslin, & Dugas, 2000). People with high levels of intolerance of uncertainty typically perceive many sources of danger in their daily lives when confronted with uncertain and/or ambiguous situations. For example, a person who is concerned that an unforeseen event could spoil his or her career might feel anxious and engage in excessive worrying about these issues as a way to respond to such uncertainties (Ladouceur et al., 2000).

Worrying, ruminating, and brooding result in chronic negative affective states that tend to deplete one's energy and ability to adaptively cope with situational challenges, which in turn exacerbates the experience of negative affect (Rozanski & Kubzansky, 2005). Thus chronic negative affect tends to be self-sustaining. In contrast, positive affect widens the array of thoughts, behaviors, and executive functioning capacities at our disposal (Fredrickson & Branigan, 2005). For example, college students who feel positive affect are less likely to perceive racial differences in faces (Johnson & Fredrickson, 2005); physicians experiencing positive affect consider more options before assigning a diagnosis (Estrada, Isen, & Young, 1997); and, during business negotiations, people in a positive mood are more likely to carefully consider divergent arguments and to reach a compromise, whereas people in more neutral states are more likely to end the bargaining period without agreement (Carnevale & Isen, 1986).

POSITIVE AFFECT

Positive affect is typically associated with approach, whereas negative affect is associated with withdrawal tendencies (Cacioppo & Berntson, 1999). Experiencing negative affect that is associated with a tendency to avoid novel and potentially dangerous situations might have been evolutionarily adaptive, because it was more costly to approach a dangerous new situation than it was to avoid a harmless novel situation. As a result, the propensity is higher to respond to negative information than to positive information. This tendency has been termed *negativity bias* (Cacioppo & Gardner, 1999).

On the flip side, avoidance tendencies immunize the members of a species from novel experiences. This is problematic if these novel situations are important for the survival of the individual or its offspring and if they thereby provide the species with an evolutionary advantage. Positive affect encourages approach behaviors and stimulates exploration and curiosity. Therefore, it is possible that the partial segregation of positive and negative affective processing is evolutionarily adaptive because it encourages the individual members of a species to explore novel situations and environments, despite the potential threat that might be associated with these situations (Cacioppo & Gardner, 1999). It follows that, from an evolutionary perspective, it is possible to experience both positive and negative affect simultaneously.

Positive affect is closely associated with subjective well-being and happiness. Subjective well-being and happiness are difficult to predict or even define, though we tend to define them in terms of people's subjective cognitive and affective evaluations of their lives (Diener, 2000). It has long been assumed that subjective well-being is a temporary state and that people can never achieve the ultimate and lasting state of happiness because their expectations rise with their possessions and accomplishments. For example, winning a million dollars in a lottery will lead to great joy, but we will eventually get used to our new luxurious lifestyle and soon compare ourselves to even richer people who live even better lives than we can afford with our lottery win. The same is true for other possessions, achievements, or accomplishments that we associate with—and even define as—*happiness*. This never-ending striving turns happiness into an elusive, dynamic, and transient state. As a result, people are stuck laboring on a "hedonic treadmill" (Brickman & Campbell, 1971); no matter how hard we try and how far we go, we can never reach the ultimate state of happiness. At the same time, unhappiness is similarly transient because people eventually adapt to situations that initially caused the unhappiness.

Closely related to happiness is *vitality*. This construct is not very well defined and researched either. Vitality has been defined as "a positive and restorative emotional state that is associated with a sense of enthusiasm and energy [and] may be considered both restorative and regenerative" (Rozanski & Kubzansky, 2005, S47). It is associated with positive affect and a general sense of joy, energy for living, and general enthusiasm (Ryan & Deci, 2000). It enhances one's concentration, intellectual performance, problem-solving ability, and willingness to take on new challenges (Fredrickson, 2000).

As already noted, it is difficult to predict happiness. Demographic characteristics (such as sex, income, education, marital status, age, and religion) contribute little to subjective well-being and happiness (DeNeve & Cooper, 1998). Subjective well-being does not change considerably with age, and men and women do not differ much in subjective well-being. Married people report being slightly happier than unmarried people. Education, occupation, and even income level are also only moderately correlated with subjective well-being. No single demographic variable can explain more than 3% of the variance in subjective well-being.

Instead, subjective well-being appears to be more closely linked to personality traits, especially those that are associated with emotional stability and tension. Furthermore, happy people tend to have strong relationships (Myers & Diener, 1995) and show hardiness and feel in control of their lives. In contrast, people with a repressive and defensive style and those who perceive events as outside of their control tend to be unhappy (DeNeve & Cooper, 1998). Many factors contribute to lasting happiness. These include the perception of living a meaningful life that is directed toward a valued goal (Emmons, 1986), being affiliated with social groups (Myers, 2000), and experiencing (Scitovsky, 1982) pleasure. I devote an entire chapter to happiness and positive affect in Chapter 7.

EMOTIONAL DISORDERS

Definition

The term *emotional disorder* is not an officially recognized diagnostic category. It is often synonymous with *affective disorders* to include the diagnoses that are subsumed under mood and anxiety disorders. The term *emotional disorder* implies that an emotion is *dis*ordered (i.e., out of order) or *ab*normal (outside the norm) because it stands out, either in relation to others or relative to the person's usual experience or functioning. But when are variations in emotional experiences normal, and when are they abnormal and disordered?

As is true for all mental disorders, emotional disorders are difficult to classify, let alone to define. Most critical for the *Diagnostic and Statistical Manual of Mental Disorders* (DSM-5; 2013) is that a condition (i.e., whatever is considered as disordered) needs to cause significant distress and/or interference with the person's life. A popular definition of a mental disorder has been offered by Jerome Wakefield (2007). According to this definition, a condition is a disorder if it is a *harmful dysfunction*. It is *harmful* because the condition causes negative consequences for the person or society, and it is a *dysfunction* because the condition prevents the person from performing a natural function as designed by evolution. For example, a fear of flying is harmful because it interferes with a person's life by complicating one's travel plans. Moreover, it is dysfunctional because avoiding air travel is not adaptive in our current society. However, McNally (2011) provided a compelling critique of this definition. He noted that a "dysfunction" cannot simply be defined by biology or evolution. Instead, values and norms influence the judgment of both dysfunction and harm. Instead of linking the term *dysfunction* to evolution, he argued that it would be more meaningful if the definition of a dysfunction were linked to a person's sociocultural background rather than the assumed evolutionary significance of a behavior, because it is often very difficult to ascertain the evolutionary significance of a behavior.

Other theorists take the relativity of mental disorders to societal context even further and question the meaningfulness of defining problems as mental disorders, unless there are clear biological correlates of the disorder. An early and vocal proponent of this position has been Thomas Szasz (1961). Szasz considers psychiatric disorders as currently defined to be arbitrary and man-made constructions formed by society with no clear empirical basis. According to Szasz, psychiatric problems, including emotional disorders such as depression and anxiety disorders, are simply labels attached to normal human experiences by society rather than medical entities. As a result, the same behaviors that are considered as an expression of an emotional disorder in one culture may be considered normal or even desirable in another culture or at another time in history. Although Szasz is correct in that psychological problems are closely linked to a person's historical and sociocultural background, it is unfounded to conclude that psychological disorders are meaningless labels without any empirical basis. The history of medicine is full of examples of disorders that show a characteristic syndrome without being able to link it to specific biological correlates. For example, early research in diabetes is a prominent example. Many years after it was defined as a syndrome, it was discovered that insulin imbalance was the cause of the disorder. Based on Szasz's strong formulation, diabetes should not have been defined as a disease entity when the cause of the illness was not yet known.

On the other extreme is the belief that emotional disorders are distinct medical entities with unique features that may be found in one's personal history or biology. For example, psychoanalytically oriented clinicians believe that emotional disorders are rooted in interpersonal conflicts, such as relationships with a parent. Based on Freudian ideas, these conflicts are typically considered to result from repression (e.g., suppression) of unwanted desires, impulses, thoughts, feelings, or wishes. More modern insight-oriented psychodynamic psychotherapists often place a relatively greater emphasis on existing or unresolved interpersonal conflicts, rather than early childhood experiences. The only problem with such psychodynamic and psychoanalytic ideas is that, even after more than 100 years, there is very little, if any, empirical support for them.

Finally, biologically oriented therapists typically believe emotional disorders are biological entities. From this perspective, mental disorders are causally linked to particular biological factors, such as dysfunctions in certain brain regions or any imbalances in certain neurotransmitters, which are molecules that transmit signals from one nerve cell to another. For example, it has been shown that the neurotransmitter serotonin is involved in feelings of anxiety and depression. Accordingly, many biologically oriented psychiatrists believe a deficiency of serotonin is the cause of many emotional disorders. More recently, researchers are trying to locate specific genes that contribute to emotional and other mental health problems (e.g., Insel & Collins, 2003)

It is not clear whether manipulating specific genes—or even neurotransmitters—can, in fact, lead to clear short-term and lasting improvements in emotional problems. Moreover, locating the biological substrate of an emotional state does not explain that emotion state. One could argue that identifying biological correlates does not provide answers because we are simply shifting the question of what causes an emotion from a psychological to a biological level. The actual "reason" for the emotional distress remains unknown (i.e., there is no heuristically useful model to explain and predict the processing and regulation of emotionally salient stimuli).

Similarly, it cannot be readily concluded that depression is caused by a deficiency in serotonin, although depression and serotonin levels are related and taking a selective serotonin reuptake inhibitor (SSRI) can help lift depression. It is clear that a "serotonin model of depression" would be overly simplistic because SSRIs do not reliably improve symptoms of depression. Furthermore, other medications that target different neurotransmitters are similarly (and moderately) effective for treating depression and other emotional disorders.

The most reasonable and empirically supported way of understanding the basis of an emotional disorder appears to be a model that considers the genetic predisposition one might have to the disorder, the societal influences that have an impact on it, and other environmental factors in its development. Emotional disorders are real and treatable problems, not simply words that are assigned to man-made and arbitrary constructs and not simply the result of an imbalance of neurochemical substances.

Diathesis–Stress Model

A variety of individual-difference factors can contribute to the development of emotional disorder. It should be noted, however, that the initiating factors (i.e., the "reasons" that emotional problems develop in the first place) are usually not the same as the reasons that the problems are maintained. Furthermore, the initiating factors are relatively unimportant for implementing effective treatment strategies because the initiating factors provide neither necessary nor sufficient information for treatment. Similarly, knowing the "reason" for a broken arm (e.g., getting in a skiing accident, getting hit by a car) is of little importance in selecting the right treatment (i.e., putting the arm in a cast). Psychological problems are certainly more complicated than a broken arm. However, the point is this: The same stressor can have different effects on different people, depending on their inherent strengths and the specific coping strategies they employ. In most cases, stressors have nonspecific effects on psychological and emotional well-being. In a small number of people, however, these stressors can lead to emotional problems, depending on their specific diatheses (i.e., vulnerabilities).

The specific diathesis of a person is primarily determined by his or her predisposition to developing a specific problem when exposed to certain stresses. This relationship is generally known as the *diathesis–stress model* of psychopathology. More recent formulations of this model identify multiple vulnerabilities. For example, in the case of anxiety disorders, Barlow (2000, 2002) formulated a triple-vulnerabilities model that includes a generalized biological and heritable vulnerability, a generalized psychological vulnerability based on early experiences in developing a sense of control over salient events, and a more specific psychological vulnerability in which one learns to focus anxiety on specific objects or situations.

The diathesis–stress model is a generally recognized theory of the development of psychological and emotional disorders. Without a diathesis, the problem might not develop in the first place. However, knowing the genetic makeup of a particular person does not tell us whether this person will or will not develop a particular disorder. The presence of a gene merely increases the likelihood of developing an emotional problem. It is estimated that there are more than 20,000 protein-coding genes in the human DNA. Which of those genes predispose some individuals to emotional problems is a task for future generations of researchers. But even if we knew the identity and combinations of those genes, it would be very difficult to predict who will and will not develop an emotional problem. In addition to the person's genetic makeup, we would need to know whether or when the person will be exposed to certain environmental influences, such as stressors, and what coping strategies the person can resort to in order to deal with the stressors.

To complicate things even further, the evolving field of epigenetics suggests that environmental experiences can lead to the expression or deactivation of certain genes. This process can lead to long-term changes in traits within an individual, traits that might also be transmitted to later generations. In other words, it appears that stressors in one generation can affect not only the emotional and psychological states of the particular person but also of his or her descendants.

Given this complexity, Barlow recently presented an elaboration and extension of the diathesis-stress model (Barlow, Ellard, Sauer-Zavala, Bullis, & Carl, 2014).This view emphasizes ongoing complex and dynamic gene–environment interactions that occur throughout the life span, offering a rich perspective to advance our understanding of the development of mental disorders, and especially neuroticism, by integrating genetic, neurobiological, and environmental contributions.

In the case of emotional disorders, we assume that a particular diathesis determines whether and how a particular external and affect-relevant event is further processed. Without this diathesis, it is highly unlikely that a person will experience an emotional disorder. The individual diathesis further determines the particular affective style the person adopts to cope with the external event. Depending on the individual's affective style, the person shows one of two general affective responses: The person either experiences predominately positive or predominantly negative affect or experiences neither one (i.e., shows blunted affect). An emotional disorder can then develop if there is insufficient positive affect and a predominance of dysregulated negative affect. It should be noted that in some cases it is also possible that a disorder will develop as a result of dysregulated positive affect (as in mania). However, it could be argued that the nature of positive affect is qualitatively different in people with mania than in healthy, happy people. The general model integrating the various influencing factors discussed earlier is summarized in Figure 2.3.

Clinical Application

Targeting emotions in therapy can improve its efficacy (Ehrenreich, Fairholm, Buzzella, Ellard, & Barlow, 2007) and guide clinical science toward innovative transdiagnostic approaches (Barlow, Allen,

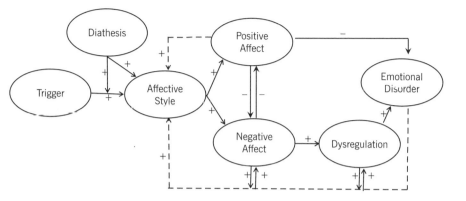

FIGURE 2.3. A diathesis–stress model of emotional disorder.

Choate, 2004; Barlow et al., 2010) that are based on sound empirical evidence rather than traditions or therapeutic orientations. More specifically, the most effective ways to treat emotional disorders, based on the model presented here, are by (1) reallocating attention to focus on events that are not emotionally distressing and promote adaptive coping; (2) modifying the affective style; (3) decreasing negative affect; (4) enhancing positive affect, which can initiate a positive cycle that is incompatible with the emotional disorder; (5) targeting affective dysregulation; (6) reexamining the context in which the emotional distress occurs; and (7) interrupting the positive feedback loops from the emotional disorder to the dysregulation of negative affect, the experience of negative affect, and affective style.

The first step when treating emotional disorders is to understand the role emotions play in a person's life. Therefore, it is important to explore the client's emotional world by conducting a thorough assessment. This is done by using guided questioning techniques, reflective listening, and empathic questioning. A "cheat sheet" for the therapist, listing examples of key questions and areas of special considerations, is given in Figure 2.4. This information will be valuable to the therapist in planning the therapy.

The following example is a dialogue between the patient, Sarah, and her therapist toward the end of the third session. Sarah's primary complaint has been severe depression. She is a 52-year-old married businesswoman with three children. Early on in treatment, it became

Components of model	Some key questions	Special considerations
External event	What is/are the events that likely triggered the emotional distress?	Consider past information to explore recurring patterns.
Diathesis	Based on the client's history, what are the vulnerability factors?	Consider the client's temperament (level of shyness), emotional granularity, alexithymia, emotional intelligence, and distress tolerance.
Affective style	What is the client's typical affective style?	Consider problem- versus emotion-focused coping and styles of emotion-focused coping. Also consider the client's emotional flexibility.
Dysregulation of negative affect	Does the client show dysregulated negative affect?	Especially consider the client's tendency to ruminate, brood, and worry.
Positive affect	What is the client's level of happiness, vitality, and quality of life?	Explore factors that negatively influence the client's positive affect and life satisfaction.

FIGURE 2.4. Therapist's cheat sheet for therapy planning.

evident that she is still struggling with her mother's death, which happened 4 years before. She had a complicated relationship with her mother, who was overly controlling. Sarah and her family decided to put her mother, who had begun suffering from dementia, into a nursing home. During the session, Sarah spontaneously expressed negative affect and provided examples of her dysregulated negative affect (inserted in the dialogue).

In Practice: Exploring Emotions

THERAPIST: Are you still thinking about your mother?

SARAH: Oh yes; every day. She is always with me.

THERAPIST: What are you feeling when you are thinking about your mother?

SARAH: I miss her a lot. I loved her very much.

THERAPIST: Did you also have any negative feelings about her?

SARAH: She was a wonderful person, but she was also pretty controlling and we often got into heated arguments. *[Expression of negative affect]*

THERAPIST: So you felt anger?

SARAH: Yes, frustration and anger at times. She also became very difficult toward the end. *[Expression of negative affect]*

THERAPIST: You loved her and you miss her and at the same time you felt anger and felt some relief when she was gone. Is this correct?

SARAH: This sounds horrible, but yes. She became difficult to take care of at the end.

THERAPIST: I can imagine. You had mentioned that she was quite demented at the end, right?

SARAH: Oh yes. Her personality changed. She was such a strong woman all her life and then became so dependent.

THERAPIST: Needy?

SARAH: Yes; needy and manipulative.

THERAPIST: Manipulative? Can you please elaborate?

SARAH: She had a way of getting what she wanted, even if this was at the expense of other people.

[Therapist explores concrete examples.]

THERAPIST: I can sense that you are having a lot of different feelings when you are thinking about your mother. Although you loved your mother, you also felt a sense of relief when she was gone. This probably causes you to feel some guilt.

SARAH: Oh definitely. I feel a lot of guilt. I am also feeling guilty because she wanted to stay with us. *[Expression of negative affect]* She hated the nursing home. But I just couldn't do it. It would have ruined my marriage. Everybody said it would be better for her to move into a nursing home.

THERAPIST: So you feel guilty because she expected to move in with you, but you sent her to the nursing home instead. *[Dysregulation of negative affect]*

SARAH: Yes.

THERAPIST: I can understand that you must have mixed emotions about your mom. There was clearly a lot of love between you. But there was also anger and frustration. Some of these feelings can cause other feelings. So the feeling of anger toward a deceased loved one can bring on feelings of guilt. So I can understand why you have such mixed feelings about your mother.

It must be quite confusing. As part of therapy, I want to help you to clarify these feelings some more. Feelings and emotions are very human, and they can be complex and complicated. It fact, it is quite normal to feel many different emotions about a person we care for deeply. There is probably not a single relationship with a person who is close to us that is simple and unidimensional. In fact, one could argue that if the emotional connection was simple and straightforward, then the relationship was probably shallow. Deep and meaningful relationships tend to cause complex emotional responses. In the first step, it will be important to recognize this complexity and to somehow come to peace with the fact that it is OK to experience also negative affect toward people we care for deeply and also for people who we love. Does it make sense what I am saying?

Given the variability between people in their emotional perception, experience, and expression, it is also important to explore existing psychological and social resources, and coping skills. This is illustrated in a later session with Sarah. The following snapshot of therapy is taken from session 5. As the therapist probed for specific coping skills, Sarah expressed many more instances when her negative affect became dysregulated.

In Practice: Exploring Emotional Health

THERAPIST: How have you been dealing with the death of your mother?

SARAH: OK, I guess.

THERAPIST: Can you tell me a bit more?

SARAH: What do you mean by dealing with her death?

THERAPIST: How are you dealing emotionally with her death? You mentioned that there were a lot of different emotions that are still present and that are still at times overwhelming. You had mentioned that you feel sadness, but also relief and a great degree of guilt. How are you dealing with these emotions?

SARAH: I am trying not to be bothered by them. *[Dysregulation of negative affect]*

THERAPIST: Bothered by what feeling in particular?

SARAH: Especially the guilt. *[Expression of negative affect]* I feel like I let her down by not moving her in with me. *[Expression of negative affect]* But everybody agreed that it would have been too difficult for me because of my mother's dementia.

THERAPIST: And perhaps some of the guilt you have today might also be related to the feeling of relief. Is this correct?

SARAH: Yes, absolutely. I loved my mother, but it became very difficult toward the end. *[Expression of negative affect]*

THERAPIST: I can imagine. What have you been doing with this feeling of guilt?

SARAH: I am trying not to feel it. *[Dysregulation of negative affect]*

THERAPIST: How do you do that?

SARAH: I am pushing the feeling away from me. *[Dysregulation of negative affect]*

THERAPIST: How else? What other strategies have you been using? Are there other family members or friends you can rely on?

SARAH: No. My sister has not been very helpful at all. And I don't really want to bother my friends with it. *[Dysregulation of negative affect]*

The brief interchange explored Sarah's existing emotional resources. It became obvious that Sarah primarily uses suppression as an emotion regulation strategy and that Sarah feels little support from other family members. She also does not believe that her friends would be an appropriate support system for her.

In sum, Sarah (1) experiences a high level of negative affect and depression; (2) experiences a low level of positive affect; (3) has problems describing and identifying her emotions; (4) typically suppresses and conceals her emotions; and (5) has difficulties adjusting and tolerating her emotions. Specific strategies to target the patient's emotional dysfunctions and dysregulations are illustrated in the following chapters.

Summary of Clinically Relevant Points

- The diathesis–stress model integrates biological, environmental, and social and psychological factors. There is a critical distinction between initiating factors (the reasons that a problem develops in the first place) and maintaining factors (the reasons that a problem persists). These factors are usually not the same, and only modifying maintaining factors can adequately treat the emotional disorders.
- The factors contributing to the diathesis include temperamental differences, emotional granularity, alexithymia, emotional clarity, emotional intelligence, and distress tolerance.

- The affective styles are interindividual differences in the habitual use of strategies to cope with emotional information. They include problem-focused versus emotion-focused strategies, different styles of emotion-focused coping, and emotional flexibility.

- Rumination, brooding, and worrying are examples of dysregulated negative affect. Together with a deficiency in positive affect, these factors lead to emotional disorders.

- Positive and negative affect interact but are not simply the opposite of one another. Positive affect involves typically relatively short, transiently energizing states that are approach-focused, whereas negative affect is an avoidant-oriented chronic feeling that often depletes one's energy, leading to a self-sustaining problem.

- The social and cultural context is important to consider for understanding and treating emotional disorders. In collectivistic societies (i.e., cultures that emphasize interdependence between its members), social contact has a greater influence on one's happiness than in individualistic societies.

CHAPTER THREE

◆

Motivation and Emotion

Motivation and emotion are closely connected. When we achieve a desired goal, we feel joy and satisfaction. In contrast, if the expected reward is not achieved, we feel frustration and anger. Because of the close association between emotions and motivations, motivation researchers have defined emotions operationally as states elicited by rewards or punishers (e.g., Rolls, 2005, 2013). A reward is anything people work for; a punisher is anything people escape from or avoid. Depending on whether a punisher or a reward is given or withheld, different emotions arise. For example, withholding a punisher elicits relief; giving a reward leads to pleasure; delivering a punisher leads to apprehension; and withholding a reward leads to frustration (Rolls, 2005).

In addition, some researchers distinguish different motivational systems that are associated with specific emotions. For example, Panksepp and Biven (2010) discuss various primary systems that are associated with positive affect, such as the seeking system, the lust system, and the play system, and other systems, such as the panic system, that are associated with negative feelings. This chapter explores in more detail the link between motivation and emotion.

THE RELATIONSHIP BETWEEN MOTIVATION AND EMOTION

In Chapter 1, I defined emotion as a multidimensional experience that is characterized by different levels of arousal and degrees of pleasure or displeasure, associated with subjective experiences and *motivational tendencies* (among other factors). Thus motivation is a part of the definition of an emotion.

However, these motivational tendencies are more obvious for some emotions than for others. Emotion and motivation are most obviously associated in mood disorders, especially depression, and addictions, such as substance use disorders, gambling, or eating disorders. Motivation can be intrinsic or extrinsic and is generally defined as a drive to act in a certain manner in order to move in a particular direction to achieve a particular goal. Intrinsic motivation refers to motivation that is driven by the person's interest and enjoyment in the activity itself, whereas extrinsic motivation depends on external desire for reward or avoidance of punishment. Goal achievement is associated with positive affect, nonachievement with negative affect. Thus motivation is causally linked to affect. Moreover, emotions can affect motivations. For example, a prospective study found that pretreatment emotion regulation skills predicted alcohol use during a psychological treatment for the use problem and that posttreatment emotion regulation skills predicted alcohol use at follow-up (Berking et al., 2011). The study further showed that it is particularly the ability to tolerate negative affect that predicts subsequent alcohol consumption.

In the case of eating disorders, ubiquitous sociocultural pressures to be thin bring about extremes in body dissatisfaction, internalization of the thin ideal promoted by the mass media, and dieting—all of which are risk factors for binge eating and bulimic behavior. Furthermore, being overweight confers risks as well. Some of these factors, including restrained eating and extreme weight and shape concerns, are addressed in cognitive-behavioral therapy, which is currently considered a first-line treatment option (Stice, 2002).

In addition, the importance of negative affectivity as a risk factor in its own right has been recognized. Specifically, a popular theory in eating disorders is the so-called *dual-pathway model of overeating.* This model assumes that negative affect and restrained eating mediate the link between body dissatisfaction and overeating (Stice, Ragan, & Randall, 2004). More specifically, the dual-pathway model proposes that restrained eating and negative affect serve as the final mechanisms by which general sociocultural pressures to be thin, as expressed by family, peers, and the media, lead to body dissatisfaction that fosters the development of eating problem behaviors, such as bulimia or overeating. The first pathway to overeating is restrained eating; the second pathway is the influence of eating on negative affect, such as depression. Dietary restraint has consistently been linked to bulimia nervosa. Together with weight concerns, shape concerns, and eating concerns, restrained eating is also a diagnostic criterion for eating disorders. Negative affect about eating is another defining criterion for eating disorders. The model assumes that people with bulimia use bingeing and purging as a means of regulating negative mood states. This model is consistent with findings showing that patients with bulimia who restrained their eating responded significantly better to cognitive-behavioral treatment than those classified mixed restraint–depressed (e.g., Stice & Agras, 1999).

An extended version of this dual-pathway model postulates that negative affect and overeating are related not directly but indirectly through lack of interoceptive awareness and emotional eating (van Strien, Engels, Leeuwe, & Snoek, 2005). More specifically, this model assumes that the link between body dissatisfaction and overeating is explained by the fact that negative affect due to body dissatisfaction is related to a lack of awareness of personal feelings and to eating while dealing with negative affect, which in turn is associated with overeating. The research literature provides empirical support for the finding that sociocultural factors are important risk factors and that negative affect predicts the maintenance of eating pathology (Koenders & van Strien, 2001; Stice, 2002).

Deficits in emotion regulation skills are also clear risk factors for maintaining mood and anxiety problems. Specifically, it has been shown that emotion regulation skills negatively and unidirectionally predict subsequent symptom severity over a 5-year period above and beyond the effects of baseline severity of depression (Berking, Wirtz,

Svaldi, & Hofmann, 2014) and anxiety (Wirtz, Hofmann, Riper, & Berking, 2014). Acceptance, tolerance, and the willingness to confront emotions had the strongest predictive effects for anxiety symptoms, whereas any skill deficit predicted symptoms of depression.

Improving these deficits also reduces emotional distress, as shown in a prospective randomized controlled trial (Berking, Ebert, Cuijpers, & Hofmann, 2013). This study assigned a large number of inpatients who met criteria for major depressive disorder (n = 432) to receive either routine cognitive-behavioral therapy or cognitive-behavioral therapy enriched with emotion regulation skills training. The results showed that patients who received the treatment with emotion regulation skills training had a significantly greater reduction in depression than the other group. Moreover, the former group of patients demonstrated a significantly greater reduction of negative affect, as well as a greater increase of well-being and emotion regulation skills particularly relevant for mental health.

MOTIVATED BEHAVIORS

Motivated behaviors are aimed at either attaining reward and pleasure or avoiding punishment and misery (e.g., Carver & Scheier, 1998; Craig, 1918; Gray & McNaughton, 2000; Mowrer, 1960). Early behaviorists directly linked affect and motivated behaviors by assuming that drive reduction is the primary mechanism of reward (Hull, 1943; Mowrer, 1960; Spence, 1956). For example, water functions as a reward because it reduces the thirst drive; food functions as a reward because it reduces the hunger drive.

Motivation theorists later rejected the notion that reward is due to drive reduction. Instead, it is assumed that hedonic reward is independent of drive reduction and that organisms are motivated by incentive expectancies, not by drive reduction (e.g., Bindra, 1974; Pfaffman, 1960; Toates, 1986; Bolles, 1972; Young, 1966). In other words, motivated behavior is a function not only of a physiological deficit but also of the learned association between a stimulus and its hedonic value. For example, refreshing drinks, tasty food, attractive sexual partners, and addictive drugs are all hedonic incentives not only because they satisfy biological drives but also because we have learned to associate these stimuli with rewarding experiences. Therefore, the sights, smells, sensations, and other cues that are associated with and predict these rewards lead a person to anticipate the rewards and so contribute to the likelihood that he or she will show motivated behaviors. Thus physiological deficits do not have to drive motivated behaviors directly.

Some rewards that are shared by virtually all animals and humans include food and water in the case of *hunger and thirst motivation* and orgasm in the case of *sexual motivation*. Humans and animals that establish social hierarchies perceive social closeness (due to *affiliation motivation*). Occupying a high level in the social hierarchy (due to *dominance motivation*) is perceived as rewarding. In addition, humans and some animals are rewarded by mastery experiences (due to *achievement motivation*), deepening a relationship to another person (due to *intimacy motivation*), and having an impact on others (due to *power motivation*) (e.g., Schultheiss & Wirth, 2008).

Many motivations are need-driven; others are primarily incentive-driven or a combination of both. For example, a period of food depletion leads to low blood sugar and the subjective experience of hunger, resulting in a strong need-driven motivation. In contrast, the chocolate mousse dessert after a five-course dinner is much more incentive-driven than need-driven. Many more complex social behaviors, such as making a marriage proposal, are likely linked to both a number of need-driven and incentive-driven motivations, ranging from sexual motivation to social affiliation and intimacy motivations. As noted earlier, emotions are in part defined by the motivational tendencies. Therefore, clarifying the motivational drive of a behavior can shed light on the emotional experience of the patients. The following example illustrates how a person's drinking motive is linked to social affiliation motivation and emotion.

In Practice: Understanding Motivations

THERAPIST: Please help me understand why you drink. What's so good about drinking?

DAVID: Well, it makes me feel good and it is part of my life. It's just what I do with John and Chuck to blow off some steam after a long day at work.

THERAPIST: So you drink to unwind and to spend time with John and Chuck.

DAVID: Yes.

THERAPIST: So drinking serves an important role in your friendship with John and Chuck, correct?

DAVID: I guess so.

THERAPIST: What would happen if you didn't drink when you get together with John and Chuck?

DAVID: This would be very awkward and would probably not be as much fun. I would probably feel like an outsider and they might wonder what is wrong with me.

THERAPIST: What would you be doing if you didn't go out drinking with John and Chuck?

DAVID: I don't know. Stay home and watch TV?

THERAPIST: And this doesn't sound good.

DAVID: No. It would be pretty depressing.

THERAPIST: Why would it be depressing?

DAVID: Because I would miss my friends.

THERAPIST: So, on the one hand, drinking helps you be with your friends. On the other hand, it also has some negative consequences, correct?

DAVID: Yes, it has gotten me into trouble.

THERAPIST: It has gotten you into trouble with your girlfriend and your boss. Plus your license got suspended for driving under the influence.

DAVID: You got it.

THERAPIST: So how did you feel when they took away your driver's license?

DAVID: Not good.

THERAPIST: And how did you feel after the fights with your girlfriend and your boss?

DAVID: Very depressed.

THERAPIST: Apparently, drinking has both positive and negative consequences. It helps you to spend some good time after work with John and Chuck, but it also leads to some serious problems with your personal life and your career, and you even got into trouble with the law. Do I understand this correctly?

DAVID: Yes.

THERAPIST: I wonder if there is way to satisfy your social need while at the same time avoiding the negative consequences of drinking. Can we brainstorm some possibilities?

David drinks alcohol to satisfy his social affiliation motive and also to relieve his depression and stress. At the same time, his drinking impairs his functioning at work and his relationship with his girlfriend. Hence, an effective treatment approach will need to address these motives that are directly linked to his depression.

APPROACH VERSUS AVOIDANCE MOTIVATION

Approaching a desirable state or object is associated with positive affect, and avoiding or escaping an undesirable object or situation reduces negative affect. Difficulties in avoiding undesirable or attaining desirable goals or objects can lead to depression, frustration, and anger. This appears to be true for all organisms, and it is particularly true for humans with their capacity to anticipate and predict future events. We experience positive affect when we anticipate future events to be pleasant and experience negative affect when we expect them to be unpleasant. The decision whether to engage in a particular behavior is, therefore, closely tied to the person's expectation of the pleasantness of the experience (Cox & Klinger, 1988).

Avoidance can be either active or passive. In the case of active avoidance, the organism actively escapes from the undesirable state or object; in the case of passive avoidance, the behavior is inhibited in order to avoid the undesirable object or state. Active avoidance may be conceived of as a form of approach motivation toward safety (e.g., Schultheiss & Wirth, 2008). For example, in the classic study by Solomon and Wynne (1953), dogs quickly learned to jump from compartment A to compartment B as soon as a stimulus (such as a light) signaling an impending foot shock in compartment A appeared. Most dogs not only learned to avoid the shock by jumping from compartment A to B within only a few trials, but this behavior also continued even if no shock was presented any longer following the light. Furthermore, the dogs showed no signs of fear once they learned how to escape the shock, suggesting that the jumping was not only motivated by active avoidance but also by approach toward safety, especially after the initial trials. This experiment also illustrates that affect is directly linked to motivation.

Depending on a person's motivational tendency, the same event or situation will be experienced very differently. For example, somebody who is highly avoidance-oriented will experience rejection or criticism differently (e.g., more strongly, for a longer time) from somebody who is more approach-oriented. Patients can enhance their understanding of their emotional experience by becoming aware of their motivational tendencies that might be associated with their emotions.

Approach motivations are closely tied to positive affective states. However, approach is not always associated with external reward and can even be experienced as a negative state (such as anger; Harmon-Jones, Harmon-Jones, & Price, 2013). For example, the *seeking* system of Panksepp and Biven's (2010) model is associated with approach motivation but does not simply respond to positive incentives. The system is also active when people (and animals) seek and find a solution to a problem or challenge. The satisfaction of finding a solution is in and of itself the rewarding and pleasurable event.

Aside from the *seeking* system, Panksepp and Biven (2010) identify a number of other systems that are part of the emotional-affective circuits in the mammalian brains. These include the fear/anxiety system, the rage/anger system, the lust/sexual system, the care/maternal nurturance system, the panic/grief separation-distress system, and the play/rough-and-tumble, physical social-engagement system. All of these systems are biologically hardwired and evolutionarily older systems that are linked to primitive emotions. For example, the fear/anxiety system allows the organism to reflexively withdraw, hide, or run away; the panic/grief system is conceived as psychological pain and is also regarded as the foundation of depression; the rage/anger system is active during acts of aggression; the lust/sexual system is active during sexual acts; the care system is active when raising offspring; and the play system is not only active when playing with offspring but is also the basis for learning and teaching social skills. These different systems can be coactivated and work synergistically. For example, the panic system, in conjunction with the care system, is assumed to lead to social bonding and social attachment.

Other theoretical accounts closely associate approach motivation with positive affect. One influential theory known as the *opponent-process theory* (Solomon & Corbit, 1974) states that all hedonic stimuli that are sufficiently strong and persist for long enough activate not just one but two responses: first, the direct hedonic response (A-process), and, second, an opponent process that is the opposite of this response (B-process). This second process is oppositely valenced to the first response. For example, if the initial hedonic response is pleasant, the opponent response is then unpleasant. This opponent process is assumed to be actively generated by the brain to all affective reactions in order to restore homeostasis and maintain a neutral affective balance. The theory, which was inspired by the sensory opponent-process theory of color vision, has been particularly influential for explaining affective states in drug addiction. The theory states that the initially reinforcing effect of the drug activates the initial A-process, leading to the positive affective A-state. The A-process then triggers the activation of the negatively valenced and opponent B-process. As a result of repeated drug use, tolerance to the drug develops, and only the negatively valenced B-state, but not the pleasant A-state, becomes more intense and longer lasting. During withdrawal, the effects of the B-state outweigh the effects of the A-state. The same principle holds true if the A-state is negatively valenced, such as in the case of pain during a long-distance run, which then later leads to the positively valenced runner's high.

Monitoring Approach and Avoidance Orientation

In order to monitor approach-versus-avoidance orientation, the therapist may ask the client to use Figure 3.1 during or between treatment sessions as a homework assignment. This form instructs the client to briefly describe a situation that elicited a strong emotional experience (e.g., having a fight with her husband) and the specific emotion she experienced (e.g., anger). The client is then instructed to indicate on a scale from 0 (*not at all*) to 100 (*very much*) whether she felt drawn toward the situation (approach-oriented) or had the desire to disengage and move away from it (avoidance-oriented). A person is approach-oriented if she feels the desire to further engage in the situation and avoidance-oriented if she feels the desire to disengage and

Instructions: Write down the date and time when you encountered a situation in which you experienced an emotion. Describe this emotion by assigning it a label (e.g., "joy" or "anger") and rate on a scale from 0 (*not at all*) to 100 (*extreme*) your desire to approach/engage with and avoid/disengage from the situation.

Date/time	Situation	Emotion label (joy, anger, etc.)	Desire to approach/ engage (0–100)	Desire to avoid/ disengage (0–100)

FIGURE 3.1. Monitoring approach and avoidance orientation.

From *Emotion in Therapy: From Science to Practice* by Stefan G. Hofmann. Copyright © 2016 by The Guilford Press. Permission to photocopy this figure is granted to purchasers of this book for personal use or use with individual clients (see copyright page for details). Purchasers can download an enlarged version of this figure (see the box at the end of the table of contents).

withdraw. Again, therapists and patients are encouraged to examine whether there is a specific pattern that is evolving.

WANTING VERSUS LIKING

The positive affective state of motivation is further separated into *wanting* versus *liking*. Wanting something is not the same as liking something. Both are kinds of reward-dependent states. *Wanting* is reward-seeking and anticipatory; *liking* is savoring and consummatory (Berridge, Robinson, & Aldridge, 2009). Wanting states and approach motivation appear to be closely associated with curiosity, as well as openness, optimism, stronger interpersonal relationships, and lower aggression. In other words, if I am craving chocolate, I am in the midst of the (pregoal) *wanting* state, searching for chocolate. Once I find a chocolate bar in the kitchen drawer and begin to eat it, I transition into the (postgoal) *liking* state. Approach motivation (wanting) typically narrows the person's attentional focus (where is the chocolate bar?) and appears to be associated with different neural circuits (Kringelbach & Berridge, 2010; Gable & Harmon-Jones 2011; Harmon-Jones, Harmon-Jones, & Price, 2013). Under normal circumstances, acquiring the things a person desires makes the person feel good. In the case of addiction, however, the *liking* and *wanting* systems can become disconnected, causing the person to continue to crave things that no longer bring pleasure, which can then lead to such compulsive behaviors as gambling, drinking, and binge eating (Robinson & Berridge, 2003).

The differentiation between liking and wanting highlights the dynamic nature of motivation. This differentiation is also consistent with earlier motivation theories that proposed that all motivated behavior can be divided into two sequential phases, an *appetitive phase* that is then followed by a *consummatory phase* (Craig, 1918). The appetitive phase consists of the flexible approach behavior that an individual engages in before the motivational goal is found, whereas the consummatory phase follows once the goal is reached. Consummatory behaviors are typically stereotypical and species-typical actions, such as licking, drinking, eating, intercourse, aggression, and so forth. It can be useful to encourage patients to distinguish the liking/consummatory phase from the wanting/appetitive phase of goals.

In Practice: Wanting versus Liking

THERAPIST: Please tell me about last weekend.

DAVID: I got totally drunk on Saturday and stayed in bed with a bad hangover most of Sunday.

THERAPIST: Did you like the time you spent in bed on Sunday?

DAVID: No, of course not. I felt miserable. My girlfriend was mad at me because we couldn't do anything together.

THERAPIST: This also happened a few weeks ago, right?

DAVID: Yes, it happened 2 weeks ago and many others times before then.

THERAPIST: So you probably knew at some point on Saturday when you were drinking that you would pay for it the next day.

DAVID: Yes.

THERAPIST: So why did you do it?

DAVID: I don't know. I guess I need to do it.

THERAPIST: Why do you think you need to drink?

DAVID: I don't know; in part because it is a social thing.

THERAPIST: So you need to do it and want to do it, but you don't like doing it. Is this correct?

DAVID: It sounds funny, but yes.

THERAPIST: Unfortunately, this is not at all unusual in people who have problems with addiction. At the beginning, drinking is fun, and you want it because you like it. But after a while, the liking becomes detached from the wanting. People who drink a lot, for example, during the day at work and maybe even in the morning, don't like doing it. In fact, some probably strongly dislike it and might feel a lot of guilt and shame around it. But they feel compelled to do it because they need it. The wanting becomes detached from the liking, tolerance to the substance develops, and the substance use problem turns into substance dependence. You might not be at this stage yet. But you will probably get to this stage unless we do something about it.

BEHAVIORAL ACTIVATION

Many emotional problems are associated with withdrawal behaviors and inactivation. As a result, people become devoid of reinforcements and pleasure, tipping the balance toward more negative and less positive affect. Behavioral activation is a relatively simple but remarkably effective method to lift a person's energy level and increase the number of positive events in his or her life, leading to greater positive affect while diminishing negative affect.

The first step in behavioral activation is to encourage the patient to keep an activity log during the week. In its simplest form, the activity log includes the time and date, location, a brief description of the activity, and a rating of how pleasant the activity was on a scale from 0 (*not pleasant at all*) to 100 (*very pleasant*). In the next step, the therapist and patient explore the reasons why some activities are pleasant and why others were rated as unpleasant. The goal is to build and increase the number of pleasant activities and to decrease the unpleasant activities and periods of inactivity during a normal week. In addition, it is desirable to establish routines in the patient's daily life and to implement regular eating and sleeping patterns. The following is an example of such an activity log.

In Practice: Activity Log

Diary for: June 15, 2015

Time	Activity	Comment and mood rating (0—low; 100—hIgh)
6:00–7:00	Woke up, got ready	10
7:00–7:30	Woke up Fred and my son, prepared breakfast and lunches	10
7:30–8:00	Had breakfast	40
8:00–9:00	Went back to bed	50
9:00–11:00	Watched TV	20
11:00–12:00	Cleaned up	10
12:00–1:00	Read paper	20
1:00–2:00	Talked to Paula	60
2:00–3:00	Went over bank statements	40
3:00–5:00	Went to store to buy groceries and run errands	20
5:00–6:00	Cooked dinner	30
6.00–7:30	Had dinner with Fred and my son	40
7:30–9:00	Watched TV	50
9:00–10:00	Argued about money	0
10:00–11:00	Got ready for bed	20

A review of this diary illustrates a number of issues: (1) the patient's mood ratings were overall low, and her highest mood rating occurred when talking to Paula; (2) the repertoire of enjoyable activities was small and ranged primarily around chores, food, and watching TV; (3) the patient's fights with her husband reliably resulted in a drop in her mood; and (4) the lowest mood ratings in general came during unstructured times and on weekends when ruminating about her life, her relationship, and her future. Finally, it was evident that the patient did not do any physical exercise.

Activity logs might help to answer some important questions such as: How withdrawn and isolated is the patient from normal daily activities? Are there adequate opportunities to experience pleasant situations? How disrupted is the patient's daily routine because of the emotional problems? Does the patient have the necessary motivation and resources to implement the behavioral strategies?

In the next step, the therapist may want to instruct the client to come up with a list of pleasant activities or tasks. The items that are on such a list depend on the patient's likes, tastes, and hobbies. Examples may include reading novels, reading and watching modern theater plays, writing novels and poetry, going for walks, playing cards with friends, and watching newly released movies.

Encouraging the patient to come up with and engage in pleasant activities can have a dramatic effect on her or his well-being. Pleasant activities tend to be self-reinforcing. The vicious cycle of inactivity, social isolation, and negative affect can be effectively disrupted by slowly and persistently introducing patients in creative ways to a range of pleasant activities. Just as behavioral inactivation and negative affect are reciprocally reinforcing, so are behavioral activation and positive affect.

These activities should be integrated gradually into the patient's homework exercises. A regular eating and sleeping routine, as well as a cardiovascular exercise routine (vigorous walking or running at least twice a week for 30 minutes each time) should be an essential part of it.

Summary of Clinically Relevant Points

- Motivation is closely tied to affect and emotions. Motivated behaviors are either approach-oriented and aimed at receiving reward and pleasure or avoidant-oriented and aimed at avoiding punishment and displeasure.

- Motivated behaviors are not only a function of physiological deficits but also a result of learned associations between the goal and the hedonic experience of the goal.

- In order to identify the associated motivational tendencies, patients may be instructed to monitor approach- and avoidance-oriented motivations associated with specific emotional states.

- Avoidance motivation can be active or passive. Active avoidance involves active escape from the undesirable state or object; passive avoidance implies that the behavior is inhibited in order to avoid the undesirable object or state.

- Approach motivation can include consummatory liking or goal-seeking wanting systems.

- Emotions are associated with the general tendency to either approach/engage with a situation or object or to avoid/disengage from a situation or object.

CHAPTER FOUR

◆

Self and Self-Regulation

Emotions, and especially emotion regulation strategies, are closely associated with what we call the *self*. In fact, some modern emotion theorists (e.g., Barrett, 2014; LeDoux, 2015) assume that the experience of emotions cannot be distinguished from self-related processes. Depending on one's level of self-control, some emotion regulation strategies will be more or less effective. Self-related processes are also closely related to affective states. We experience positive affect if we feel good about ourselves and negative affect if we feel bad about ourselves. This requires self-consciousness, self-awareness, the ability to shift perspectives, and the ability to be self-reflective.

What is the "self?" Is there only one self, or are there many different selves, depending on the situational context, other people, and one's personal history? What is "consciousness," and what are "self-consciousness" and "self-awareness"? Why are these constructs so closely tied to emotions, and how can we enhance clinical practice based on self-related processes? These are the guiding questions of this chapter.

STRUCTURE OF THE SELF

William James devoted an entire chapter in his book *Principles of Psychology* (1890/1983) to the issue of the self. He began his discussion of the subject with the observation that the process of self-awareness implies that the self is both object and subject—an aspect that *needs to be known* and an aspect that *knows* (i.e., that is the knower). He referred to these discriminated aspects as the *Me* (object, which is the aspect that is known) and the *I* (the subject, which is the aspect that is the knower).

To further elaborate on this distinction, James identified various characteristics of the *I*-self and parts, or constituents, of the *Me*-self. The characteristics of the *I*-self include self-awareness (an appreciation of one's internal states, needs, thoughts, feelings), self-agency (the sense of authorship over one's actions and thoughts), self-continuity (the sense that one remains the same person over time), and self-coherence (the sense that the self is a stable, single, and coherent entity). The constituents of the *Me*-self include the *material Me*, the *social Me*, and the *spiritual Me*. Examples of the *material Me* are the body, the clothes, and the things we possess. The *social Me* is determined by the recognition one gets from one's peers. Because there are a multitude of different social groups and individuals associated with an individual, James assumed that there are also a multitude of different social Me's. Finally, the *spiritual Me* is determined by one's metaphysical beliefs and relationship to God. James placed different values on these Me's and arranged them in a hierarchy, with the material Me at the bottom, the spiritual Me at the top, and the social Me in between.

Many influential writers after James explored the structure and characteristics of the self. Some authors described the self as a unitary construct and examined the different characteristics that describe these different aspects of the self. For example, Allport (1955) defined the self as those aspects of personality that the person considers central to his or her own personality. Other writers described it as a construct consisting of those characteristics of a person that are stable rather than unstable (Snygg & Combs, 1949) and that a person is aware of and has control over (Rogers, 1951).

Cooley (1902) defined the self as consisting of whatever characteristics were associated with first-person pronouns ("I am . . . "). It was assumed that the person perceives him- or herself the way others do, and this was referred to as the *looking-glass self.* Thus each person consists of as many selves as there are significant others in his or her social life. This view places a greater emphasis on *social consciousness* (i.e., awareness of others and society) as opposed to *self-consciousness.* Social consciousness involves awareness of how the significance of a person's action is determined by the reactions of others. Similarly, Mead (1934) and Sarbin (1952) posited that a person has as many selves as there are social roles for this individual. Sarbin (1952) further proposed that everybody possesses a number of *empirical selves* that correspond to the different social roles that we are expected to occupy. The *pure ego* is the cross-section of these different empirical selves. Similarly, Gergen (1971) argued that we possess multiple selves corresponding to our multiple social identifications.

To sum up this brief historical review, the self is generally viewed as a multidimensional construct consisting of global and domain-specific self-evaluations, which are represented as hierarchical and dynamic schemas and structures.

SELF-AWARENESS

Self-awareness—the awareness of the existence of one's self—is not unique to humans, and it is closely tied to empathy and social intelligence (which is also apparent in some nonhuman primates, such chimpanzees). The term *social intelligence* refers to the competitive maneuvering for scarce resources using the social structure (Humphrey, 1976). This viewpoint was based on laboratory tests, in which primates appear to be much more intelligent than they would need to be in order to accomplish everyday problems that they face in nature, such as finding food and protecting against predators. Therefore, it was hypothesized that the driving force behind the evolution of primate intelligence was not recognizing, memorizing, and processing of any specific skills. Rather, it was the social interaction of these animals and the ability to recognize the members of one's social group, deceive one another, track relationships, and so forth that required the necessary brain power. The recognition that it is adaptive for members of a species to predict and manipulate the minds of other members, together with empirical support from field observations of nonhuman primates (Jolly, 1966), led to the *social intelligence hypothesis* and the *theory of mind* concept. Consistent with this concept were observational studies in chimpanzees (Goodall, 1971; de Waal, 1982) and baboons (Byrne & Whiten, 1985) showing behaviors that indicate tactical deception. An example is a case of a juvenile male baboon who distracted an older and dominant male to avoid a fight by using such deception. Although no predator was in fact approaching, the juvenile male pretended that he noticed great danger by displaying a typical gesture that involves standing on his hind legs and looking attentively into the distance. As a result, the dominant older male stopped his attack and prepared himself for an approaching predator that never came.

These observations raise important questions about the uniqueness of the self in humans, because they suggest that self-awareness exists in nonhuman primates. For example, chimpanzees spontaneously learn to use a mirror to explore parts of themselves that they had never had the opportunity to examine before, such as their own face, teeth, or their anus (Gallup, 1970, 1979). Moreover, chimpanzees have been shown to recognize themselves in the mirror (Gallup, 1970). Aside from humans, only a few primate species (chimpanzees, orangutans, and some others) share the ability to recognize themselves in a mirror.

A construct closely related to self-awareness is *self-consciousness*, which is generally believed to involve attention and monitoring in addition to awareness. Some authors emphasize the importance of distinguishing self-description from self-evaluation of private versus public aspects of self-consciousness (e.g., Fenigstein, Scheier, & Buss, 1975; Harter, 1999). For example, self-evaluations are judgments about one's own competence or adequacy, and they can be either about private aspects of the self (e.g., "I have a short fuse") or public aspects of the self (e.g., "I have nice hair"). Similarly, self-statements can either relate to private characteristics of a person (i.e., those aspects that are related to private self-consciousness) or to public aspects of the self (i.e., those aspects that are related to public self-consciousness).

People base their self-worth partly on their social roles and relationships with other people (Markus & Kitayama, 1991), and the perceptions of the opinions of others toward the self are important determinants of self-perception (Cooley, 1902; Mead, 1925). Therefore, self-perception includes, at a minimum, judgments about one's competence, bodily appearance, and personality characteristics that can be either socially relevant or not socially relevant.

Assessment techniques of self-evaluation have primarily employed self-report measures that require individuals to indicate whether they view themselves positively or negatively in various domains (e.g., Fenigstein et al., 1975). Methodologies that focus on self-description ask respondents to define themselves in response to the question *Who am I?* (e.g., Harter, 1999). This technique lends itself to a content analysis of spontaneously generated self-statements that are coded into different categories to isolate the dimensions that are most salient to the individual's self-representation. However, the distinction between self-description and self-evaluation can be blurry and arbitrary. In addition, as already discussed, self-perception is situation-dependent.

Previous experiments on self-perception have used the presence of a mirror to enhance self-focused attention (e.g., Duval & Wicklund, 1972; Hofmann & Heinrichs, 2002). For example, we have employed mirror manipulation in combination with a forced-choice self-statement technique to investigate the differential effect of heightened self-focused attention on self-perception and self-evaluation in a group of undergraduate students (Hofmann & Heinrichs, 2002). In this study, we asked participants to write down three positive and three negative aspects of themselves. Before completing this task, half of the participants sat in front of a large mirror for 5 minutes. The students' self-statements were classified into one of the following categories: (1) bodily appearance; (2) competence; (3) socially relevant personality characteristics (e.g., "I am competitive" or "I am a good friend"); (4) non-socially relevant personality characteristics (e.g., "I am a procrastinator" or "I am creative"); and (5) "other" (for statements that did not fit into any of the other categories). The results showed that the presence of a mirror has a moderating effect on self-evaluation and leads to more statements about public aspects and to fewer self-critical statements about private aspects of the self.

DEVELOPMENT OF THE SELF

Humans develop self-recognition in a mirror by about 18–24 months (Brooks-Gunn & Lewis, 1984). This is also the time when children form relations between objects and events around them and cognitive schemas. Therefore, it is possible that the contingency between the self-actions (i.e., the behavior of the child) and seeing these actions in the mirror triggers the formation of an equivalency relation between the individual's internal self-representation and the external stimuli as seen in the mirror (i.e., the child's action being reflected in the mirror; Povinelli, 1995).

The social context for the developing self becomes especially important between the ages of 3 and 6, when social regulation evolves. Social regulation then becomes a fundamental aspect of human socialization. This is the time when the child starts to respond based on other people's inner states rather than to their outward behaviors and learns as well to relate the present self (who I am now) to the past self (who I was then), as well as the future self (who I will be; Higgins & Pittman, 2008).

SELF AND AFFECT

Self-focused attention has been described as a specific form of cognitive bias that is strongly related to negative affect (Ingram, 1990; Mor & Winquist, 2002). An earlier review of the literature suggested that negative self-focus is a general factor of psychopathology with specific kinds of self-relevant information being disorder-specific and reflecting the particular psychopathological schemas of the various disorders. According to this view, self-focused attention can become maladaptive if the person is unable to shift to an external focus of attention when the situation warrants; this leads to self-absorption (an excessive, sustained, and inflexible attention to internal states; Ingram, 1990).

In contrast, Pyszczynski and Greenberg (1987) noted that Ingram's (1990) model might overestimate the extent of the relationship between self-focus and various pathological conditions, other than depression. These authors proposed that depression specifically is associated with negative self-focused attention. More specifically, the authors suggested that depression is a consequence after the loss of an important source of self-worth, when a person becomes stuck in a self-regulatory cycle without being able to reduce the discrepancy between actual and desired states. The model assumes that the person then falls into a pattern of continuous self-focus, leading to negative affect, self-perception, and preferential focus on negative over positive outcomes. A more recent review suggests that private self-focus was relatively more strongly associated with depression and generalized anxiety, whereas public self-focus was more strongly associated with social anxiety (Mor & Winquist, 2002).

The concept of self-focus was also a central component in an early self-regulation model (Duval & Wicklund, 1972). According to this model, self-focused attention leads to a self-evaluative process in which a person's current state in a particular self-relevant domain is compared with his or her standard in that domain. The model states that the person experiences positive affect if the current standing surpasses the standard, whereas negative affect is experienced if the current standing falls short of the standard. The experience of negative affect then leads to attempts to decrease the discrepancy or to avoid self-focus. Building on this model, Carver and Scheier (1998) proposed that self-focus plays an important role in the self-regulatory processes toward goal pursuit by allowing the person to gather information about the discrepancy between his or her current self and a salient standard and engage in discrepancy-reducing behaviors when a negative discrepancy is detected. The model states that if there is a match between the current self and the desired standard, the person terminates the regulatory process. In contrast, if the current self falls short of the standard, the person is assumed to enter a cycle of behaviors and evaluations that lasts until the self matches the standard or until the person determines that a match is impossible. Negative affect is experienced as a result of individuals' judgment that the likelihood of attaining the standard is low or if the progress toward one's goals would be too slow.

The future self is obviously closely associated with one's values, goals, and ideals. Therefore, self-regulation involves making decisions in the present in relation to future goals (Carver & Scheier, 1998). If the consequences of these decisions are congruent with these goals, standards, and values, the self is perceived as positive; if they are incongruent, the self is perceived as negative (Higgins, 1987). For example, if people experience a discrepancy between their present state (*actual self*) and the type of person they hope or aspire to be (*ideal self*), they feel discouraged, sad, and depressed, and their willingness to engage in a task is weakened. If people experience a discrepancy between their present state and the type of person they believe they have to become (*ought self*), they worry, feel anxiety, and are nervous, and their engagement and vigilance in tasks increases (Higgins, 1987). In contrast, people have positive affect toward themselves if they become the type of persons they value becoming.

Thus Higgins's self-discrepancy theory (e.g., Higgins, 1987) posits that emotions are not a direct product of any specific behavioral outcome. Rather, emotions are seen as a product of the perceived discrepancy between the desired state and the present state. If there is such a discrepancy, conditional thoughts occur. These conditional thoughts take the form of *if–then* statements (e.g., "if I had done X, Y would have happened"). The tendency of people to imagine alternatives to reality is called *counterfactual thinking* (e.g., Mandel, Hilton, & Catellani, 2005; Roese, 1997). People experience affect when there is a discrepancy between an actual outcome and a salient ideal alternative outcome (Epstude & Roese, 2008). This affective contrast can lead to negative or positive mood, depending on the type of counterfactuals. For example, positive affect may be experienced by imagining less desirable alternatives (e.g., "if I had married my first girlfriend, I would have been divorced by now"). Such thinking can reduce negative affect or maintain positive affect.

Kendall and Hollon (1981) introduced the term *power of nonnegative thinking* for the phenomenon that the absence or reduction of negative self-referential thoughts is more relevant to psychopathology than the presence or increase of positive thoughts. One possible method for relating positive and negative thoughts is the *states of mind* (SOM) model (Schwartz, 1986, 1997). This model quantifies the valence of thoughts by relating positive thoughts (P) to the sum of positive and negative (N) thoughts [P/(P + N)]. Specific values of SOM ratios are associated with certain information-processing characteristics. Initially, Schwartz (1986) proposed five distinct SOMs, with the most adaptive cognitive state reflected by a balance of positive and negative thoughts. This balance appears to be associated with an SOM ratio of 0.62 or higher (i.e., at least 62% of positive self-statements; Schwartz & Garamoni, 1989). Schwartz (1997) later reformulated the SOM and included seven qualitatively different categories. In this revised model, the most adaptive cognitive state (*positive dialogue*) is divided into three subcategories: *superoptimal* (0.85–0.90), *optimal* (0.78–0.84), and *normal* (0.67–0.77). The SOM ratio of 0.62 is in the *successful coping dialogue* category of the revised SOM model.

The model assumes that the more the ratio deviates from the positive dialogue, the higher the degree of psychopathology is. If positive cognitions are extremely overrepresented (> 0.90; *positive monologue*), it is assumed that the individual has lost his or her attentiveness to threatening events. A conflicted dialogue is a state in which positive and negative information are equally salient in an individual's mind (0.42–0.58) and is usually associated with mild levels of anxiety and/or depression. A *failed coping dialogue* (0.34–0.41) is associated with moderate depression or anxiety, and a *negative dialogue* (0.10–0.33) is associated with severe depression or anxiety. A *negative monologue* is defined as an SOM ratio of below 0.10 and indicates extreme negativity in cognitive contents that is usually associated with severe psychopathology (Schwartz, 1997).

Self-determination theory (Ryan & Deci, 2000) similarly highlights the strong connection between the self and affect. This theory suggests that an open awareness is especially beneficial in facilitating the choice of behaviors that are consistent with one's values, needs, and interests. In contrast, mindless and automatic processing can negatively affect considerations of options that are more congruent with one's needs and values (Ryan, Kuhl, & Deci, 1997). To be more precise, although automaticity saves time and frees one's mind for more important tasks, it can also have negative consequences if deployment of conscious attention overrides unwanted responses and if such deployment is linked to well-being in cognitive, emotional, and behavioral domains (Bargh & Ferguson, 2000; Baumeister, 2015).

Self-Control

Self-control is the person's ability to control his or her emotions and behavioral impulses. Being able to delay gratification and to control our initial impulses in order to modulate our emotional experience and expression promotes mental and physical health, as well as overall adjustment in society.

Self-control, which is associated with executive functioning and activation in the frontal cortices, has been shown to be under the influence of both genetics and environment (Bouchard, 2004; Epstein, 2006). Deficits in self-control predict early mortality (Kern & Friedman, 2008); psychiatric disorders (Caspi, Moffitt, Newman, & Silva, 1996); unhealthy behaviors such as overeating, smoking, unsafe sex, drunk driving, and noncompliance with medical regimens (Bogg & Roberts, 2004); and delinquency (White et al., 1994). For example, it has been shown that 4-year-old children who delayed gratification longer in certain situations developed into more cognitively and socially competent adolescents, achieving higher scholastic performance and coping better with frustration and stress (Mischel, Shoda, & Rodriguez, 1989). Self-control can be reliably assessed by giving a 4-year-old child a marshmallow and telling the child that he or she can eat it anytime he or she wants; however, if the child waits 15 minutes, he or she will receive another marshmallow. It has been shown that the child's ability to delay gratification was associated with later success, as well as cognitive and social competence later in life.

These findings are consistent with other, longitudinal research, such as the longitudinal study conducted in Dunedin, New Zealand. This study followed up 1,000 children from birth to age 32 (Moffitt et al., 2011). The results showed that differences in self-control in childhood predicted physical health and substance dependence, as well as personal finances and even criminal behaviors. The same study also showed that in a sample of 500 sibling pairs, the sibling with lower self-control had more emotional and behavioral problems, despite growing up in the same family. This study assessed self-control by observing the child's behaviors, such as lability, low frustration tolerance, hostility, roughness, resistance, restlessness, impulsivity, inattention, and lack of persistence. Children with poor self-control were at higher risk for developing substance dependence later on in life. Children with poor self-control were also more likely to struggle financially in adulthood, and they were more likely to be convicted of a criminal offense, even after accounting for social class and IQ. In summary, these studies demonstrate that difficulties with controlling one's emotions and impulses are associated with poor physical, psychological, and social adjustment. Longitudinal studies further suggest that these difficulties are apparent at a very early age and appear to be relatively stable personality traits.

Affective Forecasting

Self-consciousness allows us to travel in time by remembering the past and anticipating the future. With *prefactual thinking*, people imagine how they will think and feel in the future about a decision that they make now (McConnell et al., 2000). People can imagine that if they were to make a particular choice now, in the future they may feel that another choice would have been better, leading to self-criticism and feelings of regret over their past decision (e.g., "if I buy the car today and find it for less next week, I'll regret my purchase").

Counterfactual thinking, prefactual thinking, and the anticipated fear of future regret influence people's decisions in the present moment (Mandel et al., 2005). In fact, people may be influenced by those thinking patterns too much because once an event has actually occurred people are less susceptible to self-criticism and regret over a negative event than they imagined beforehand that they might be (Gilbert, 2006). Research on *affective forecasting* (i.e., people's predictions of their future feelings if particular events were to happen) showed that people tend to overestimate the intensity of the pleasure and positive affect or displeasure and negative affect they will feel when an event occurs (e.g., winning $1 million in a lottery or the death of one's spouse) and also to overestimate how long the pleasure or displeasure will last after the event (Gilbert, 2006). One important reason that people mispredict is that they tend to overestimate the impact of an event on their emotions and underestimate the self-regulatory processes that attenuate them. Another important reason for such mispredictions is *focalism*, which is the tendency in the present to have in mind only the focal to-be-predicted event and not to consider the surrounding circumstances that will co-occur with that event in the future (Wilson, Wheatley, Meyers, Gilbert, & Axsom, 2000).

One technique to reduce the effect of focalism is to have people focus on and imagine not just a single future event (e.g., lying on the beach after moving to California to take a new job) but also all of the surrounding circumstances and factors that would contribute to their affective state in the future (e.g., the fact that the job is with a computer company in Silicon Valley in a stressful work environment that will allow little time for anything else; Wilson et al., 2000).

In Practice: Predicting Emotions in the Future

THERAPIST: I would like to talk a little bit about your worries about your husband's job. What are you concerned about?

LAUREN : I am concerned that he will get laid off and not be able to find another job. He is making good money as a programmer and we rely on this.

THERAPIST: What are you afraid would happen if he did lose his job?

LAUREN: Well, we need his income to pay for rent and living expenses, not to mention our college debt.

THERAPIST: What would happen if you did not have the money to pay for all of that?

LAUREN: Well, we do need the money to pay for this all. We would first use up our savings and then I don't know.

THERAPIST: So what if all the money was gone? What would happen then?

LAUREN: Wow. This is a scary thought. We would end up being homeless and live on the street.

THERAPIST: And what would happen to your marriage?

LAUREN: I would stand by my husband. But I think this would be an enormous stress on our relationship.

THERAPIST: And the stress could be too high for the relationship to survive.

LAUREN: Yes. We would probably have to split up and go our own ways.

THERAPIST: What do you think is the likelihood that that you end up on the street, separated from your husband, if he loses his job?

LAUREN: This is a very scary thought and I hope that it is not going to happen. I really don't want to think about it.

THERAPIST: I understand. It is a very disturbing thought. It would be very helpful if we could talk for just a little bit longer about this. Would this be OK?

LAUREN: Sure.

THERAPIST: How do you think you would feel if your husband lost his job and there was no prospect for him of finding another job as a programmer?

LAUREN: It would be horrible. I would be devastated.

THERAPIST: Interestingly, there is a good chance you would not feel as bad as you think you would feel. Research has shown that people reliably overestimate how badly they will feel if a particular dreaded event actually does happen. Research in this field is called affective forecasting. You will also probably overestimate today how good you would feel if you won one million dollars in the lottery tomorrow. There are many reasons for this phenomenon. One of the reasons is because we tend not to take other factors into consideration, including our natural coping skills. Have you experienced situations in the past when you anticipated that something bad was going to happen, but when it did happen you did not feel as bad as you thought you would feel?

SELF, RUMINATION, AND WORRYING

Several theorists have addressed the contributions of rumination and negative self-related processes to emotional disorders, especially depression. It should be noted that, consistent with other authors (e.g., Nolen-Hoeksema, 2000), I define rumination as a maladaptive and repetitive cognitive and often verbal process, typically about past events, often associated with negative self-related processes and usually with negative affect. Simply thinking about past events is an example of recollection and reflection. Unlike rumination, reflection is not typically associated with negative affect.

Rumination and self-focused attention show some common but also unique features. Rumination has been defined as thoughts that focus the person's attention on the depressed mood and the possible causes and consequences of this mood state (Nolen-Hoeksema, Morrow, & Fredrickson, 1993), causing the person to have greater negative affect and preventing the individual from engaging in adaptive coping strategies.

A cognitive process related to rumination is worry. Both worry and rumination are repetitive thought styles that are closely correlated (Watkins, 2004). Worrying has been primarily examined in relation to anxiety (e.g., Borkovec et al., 1998), whereas rumination has been most closely studied in the context of depression (Nolen-Hoeksema & Davis, 1999). Rumination refers to the tendency to focus on the causes and consequences of problems without moving into active problem solving (e.g., Nolen-Hoeksema, 2000). In contrast, worrying appears to be an attempt to prevent or minimize future problems and might act as a cognitive avoidance strategy to reduce negative affect associated with intrusive catastrophic images (Borkovec et al., 1998). A number of recent empirical studies support this distinction (e.g., Fresco, Frankel, Mennin, Turk, & Heimberg, 2002; Segerstrom, Stanton, Alden, & Shortridge, 2003).

Worrying is a maladaptive, future-oriented cognitive process about a potential threat. As the threat becomes more imminent, worry can shift to anticipatory anxiety and later possibly to fear and panic, which are associated with greater autonomic arousal (Craske, 1999). Worrying is associated with thinking about a problem that is rather vague and not overly concrete, which leads to reduced imagery and provides insufficient strategies toward a problem solution (Davey, 1994; Davey, Jubb, & Cameron, 1996; Stöber & Borkovec, 2002). It has been associated with reduced autonomic flexibility as a result of low cardiac vagal tone (Borkovec & Hu, 1990; Hoehn-Saric & McLeod, 2000; Lyonfields, Borkovec, & Thayer, 1995; Thayer, Friedman, & Borkovec, 1996). For example, Thayer et al. (1996) showed that, relative to baseline and relaxation conditions, experimentally induced worrying was associated with higher heart rate but lower high-frequency spectral power, which is an indicator of cardiac vagal tone.

This inhibitory effect of worrying on cardiovascular activity was nicely demonstrated in a study by Borkovec and Hu (1990). In this study, a group of undergraduate students with speech anxiety, while being measured for changes in heart rate response from baseline, were instructed to engage in relaxed, neutral, or worrisome thinking just prior to visualizing a public speaking situation. Participants in the worry group displayed less heart rate response than those in the neutral condition, who showed less response than those who engaged in relaxation prior to the phobic imagery. Other research also shows that worrying is typically associated with greater anxiety and greater left-frontal alpha electroencephalography (EEG; e.g., Hofmann et al., 2005). A more detailed discussion of the neurobiology of emotions is presented in Chapter 8.

Studies investigating cognitive processes often distinguish between verbal thoughts and visual images. These two cognitive phenomena seem to have very different effects on the psychophysiological response to emotional material. For example, verbalizing a fearful situation typically induces less cardiovascular response than visually imagining the same situation (Vrana, Cuthbert, & Lang, 1986), possibly because verbalizations are used as a strategy for abstraction and disengagement in order to decrease sympathetic arousal to aversive material (Tucker & Newman, 1981). This suggests that the verbal activity during worrying is less closely connected to the affective, physiological, and behavioral systems than images are and might therefore be a poor vehicle for processing emotional information (Borkovec et al., 1998).

Research points to different subtypes of anxiety with different biological markers (Gruzelier, 1989; Heller, Nitschke, Etienne, & Miller, 1997; Nitschke & Heller, 2002). More specifically, it has been hypothesized that the left hemisphere is more involved when there are strong verbal and cognitive components associated with the anxious emotional state, such as with worrying (Heller et al., 1997). In contrast, the right hemisphere is assumed to be more involved during anticipation of imminent threat. Specifically, Heller and colleagues (1997) distinguish between *anxious apprehension* and *anxious arousal*. Anxious apprehension is defined as a state of anxiety characterized predominantly by verbal and cognitive components and directed toward future negative events. In contrast, the state of *anxious arousal* is characterized primarily by a somatic fear response and heightened physiological arousal. The authors found relatively greater right parietal activation during anxious arousal and larger frontal asymmetry in favor of the left hemisphere during a task designed to induce anxious apprehension.

Worrying processes are effectively targeted by converting the verbal thought into a concrete image, such as a scene or picture. This image can serve as a symbol of the underlying concern that then creates the specific emotional experiences.

In Practice: Worry Exposure

THERAPIST: Now let's create an image in our minds; a very ugly image of this worst-case scenario. Your husband lost his job, he was unable to find a new job, you used up all of your savings. You separated from him and you live alone on the street. Please imagine a particular scenario or picture. What do you see?

LAUREN: I am sitting on the sidewalk, begging people for money.

THERAPIST: Tell me as many details of this image as possible.

LAUREN: It's hot. I am sweating. People are walking by, ignoring me.

THERAPIST: Great job! So you're sweating and smelling of sweat because it is hot and you had not taken a shower in weeks. You are abandoned and lonely. Please close your eyes now and picture this scene as vividly as you can. If you have distracting thoughts or a desire to push this image away, simply acknowledge this desire but gently refocus on the image again. Experience the feeling that the image creates without trying to make it better. Please keep your eyes closed and stay in this situation for a few minutes. I will tell you when you can open your eyes again.

After this exercise, the therapist may ask Lauren to rate her level of discomfort on a 0 (*no discomfort*) to 100 (*very strong discomfort*) scale. The practice is likely to create high discomfort (i.e., 60 or greater). If the level of discomfort is milder, the therapist should explore the reasons for it. It is not unlikely that the patient uses experiential avoidance strategies to modulate the level of distress. Such avoidance strategies need to be eliminated by stressing the importance of fully experiencing the feeling in order to learn alternative strategies to deal with these emotions.

Summary of Clinically Relevant Points

- Self-related processes (self-awareness, self-consciousness, and self-focused attention) lead to self-perception and self-evaluations that can be positive or negative and associated with negative affect. The clinician can access the client's perception of the self by asking him or her to describe him- or herself (e.g., "I am . . . ").

- The self changes with time. The *actual self* is the self the person him- or herself is in the current state; the *ideal self* is the self one wants to be; the *ought self* is the self the person thinks others want him or her to be. A discrepancy between the *actual self* and the *ideal self* can lead to depression; a discrepancy between the *actual self* and the *ought self* can lead to stress and anxiety.

- People use strategies to protect the self. Some of these self-protective strategies include counterfactual thinking (imagining outcomes of alternative behaviors that could have been made in the past) and prefactual thinking (anticipated feeling in the future about a decision being made in the present).

- People tend to overestimate the intensity of positive and negative affect they think they will experience if a particular event happens because people underestimate the importance of self-regulatory processes and because people tend not to consider the surrounding circumstances that will co-occur with that event in the future (which is known as *focalism*).

- Self-control is the ability to delay gratification by controlling one's emotions and impulses in order to receive future rewards. Poor self-control is associated with poor psychological, physical, and social adjustment.

- Rumination and worrying are maladaptive cognitive processes that involve self-related processes leading to negative affect. Rumination is typically focused on past events, whereas worrying is typically focused on the future. Both thinking styles tend to be repetitive verbal processes rather than images, to show a low level of concreteness, and to lead to few effective problem solutions.

CHAPTER FIVE

◆

Emotion Regulation

Although emotions appear to happen automatically, we do have at least some control over our emotional experience. We can avoid the situations, people, or triggers that elicit emotional responses from us in the first place; we can refuse to allow an emotion to upset us; or we can change our view of the situation that sparked the emotion. Other important aspects that determine our emotional experience include our expectations and the context in which an emotion occurs.

The experience of an emotion can be private. At other times, we seek human contact to make us feel better or to enhance our emotional experience. Therefore, emotion regulation involves both intrapersonal and interpersonal processes. This chapter discusses the many ways in which emotions can be controlled and regulated. I examine both intrapersonal emotion regulation strategies (i.e., strategies that are relatively independent of the social context) and interpersonal emotion regulation strategies (i.e., strategies that involve other people).

DEFINING EMOTION REGULATION

Compared with animals, humans are highly skilled at regulating their emotions in order to adjust their behavior to the situational demands. This skill appears to be evolutionarily adaptive (e.g., Davidson, 2003; Ekman, 2003; Izard, 1992; Lazarus, 1991) and is closely associated with cognitive appraisal processes that distinguish humans from nonhumans (e.g., Frijda, 1986; Gross & John, 2003; Lazarus, 1991; Scherer & Ellgring, 2007). Thompson (1994, pp. 27–28) offered the following definition of emotion regulation:

> *Emotion regulation consists of the extrinsic and intrinsic processes responsible for monitoring, evaluating, and modifying emotional reactions, especially their intensive and temporal features to accomplish one's goals.*

This definition considers emotion regulation as a broad construct that includes a number of loosely associated processes, rather than a unitary concept. More specifically, this definition suggests that: (1) emotion regulation can involve maintaining, enhancing, and inhibiting emotions; (2) emotion regulation influences a number of aspects of the emotional experience, including its valence, intensity, and temporal features; (3) emotions are not only modified through self-regulation strategies but can also be regulated by others; (4) emotion regulation involves a function (i.e., emotions are regulated for a reason and are directed toward a goal). Building on this conceptualization, Gross (2002) defined emotion regulation as the process by which people influence which emotions they have, when they have them, and how they experience and express these emotions.

EMOTION REGULATION AND COPING

The recent literature on emotion regulation is closely related to the much older literature on coping. Coping is defined as the cognitive and behavioral effort to manage stressors (Lazarus, 1966, 1981, 2000; Lazarus & Folkman, 1984). There are two primary coping strategies: problem-focused (those intended to change the stressful situation) and emotion-focused (those intended to regulate one's response to the stressor). These two strategies can be employed individually or simultaneously (Lazarus & Folkman, 1984).

Stress is difficult to define. Early accounts defined stress as a stimulus or agent that places demands on the organism or as a response of the organism to particular stimuli. Other theorists distinguished the *stressor* from the *stress reaction*, whereby the *stressor* refers to the external event and eliciting stimulus and *stress reaction* to the response to the stimulus (Frydenberg, 1997; Lazarus, 2000). A useful strategy for lowering stress is to apply relaxation techniques, such as progressive muscle relaxation (see Appendix II). Clients who experience high levels of stress often benefit from using this technique on a regular basis. Regular physical exercise is similarly beneficial for coping with stress.

An integrative model of stress was proposed by Lazarus (e.g., 1966). In this model, Lazarus defined stress as a dynamic transaction between the person and the environment, which is appraised by the person as taxing or exceeding his or her resources and endangering his or her well-being. This transactional cognitive-mediational model emphasizes cognitive appraisal as a crucial component of stress. The model posits that stressful events are perceived as demanding after an initial cognitive appraisal. Thus a particular situation is not *stressful* per se, but it is the subjective appraisal of it as being challenging or otherwise demanding that makes the stimulus or event stressful. Other important contributing factors include the beliefs about the accessibility of adequate coping skills to deal with these stressful challenges. Moreover, variations in personality characteristics modulate these appraisals and responses (e.g., Lazarus, DeLongis, Folkman, & Gruen, 1985).

The model assumes that maladaptation is not a result of the stress alone but is a result of the interaction between the environment and the person's vulnerabilities and available resources. These person variables determine the individual's *coping style*, which is the habitual way of responding to stress (Lazarus & Folkman, 1984). Whereas coping is seen as a conscious and purposeful process, *coping styles*, which grew out of the psychoanalytic tradition, are believed to be largely unconscious in nature. Therefore, the ultimate choice and sequence of coping processes are not only determined by the appraisal of the situation (whether it can be changed and/or mastered) but also by the resources the individual believes he or she has (such as health, personality traits, beliefs about personal control and skills, social support, and material resources) and personal and environmental constraints that may thwart coping efforts or necessitate the use of alternative strategies (Lazarus & Folkman, 1984).

INTRAPERSONAL EMOTION REGULATION

Emotion-focused coping strategies, as defined by Lazarus and colleagues (e.g., Lazarus & Folkman, 1984), include the emotion regulation strategies as defined by Gross (2002). This intrapersonal emotion regulation model has had a significant influence on clinical research (for a review, see Gross, 2013). The model assumes that emotions can be regulated at various stages in the process of emotion generation: (1) selection of the situation, (2) modification of the situation, (3) deployment of attention, (4) modification of cognitive appraisal, and (5) modulation of responses. Emotion regulation strategies can be broadly distinguished into *response-focused* and *antecedent-focused* strategies, depending on the timing during the process that generates an emotion. Antecedent-focused emotion regulation strategies occur before the emotional response has been fully activated. They include tactics such as situation modification, attention deployment, and cognitive reframing of a situation. Suppression is a response-focused emotion regulation strategy that entails attempts to alter the expression or experience of emotions after response tendencies have been initiated.

The term *antecedent-focused strategy* might be a misnomer because it suggests that a person uses strategies *before* an emotion arises. It is more accurate to assume that some strategies are used at an *early stage* to dampen the intensity or modify the quality of an emotion rather than to prevent the experience of an emotion in the first place.

In typical experiments to examine intraindividual emotion regulation strategies (e.g., Gross, 1998a, 1998b), healthy participants are asked to view pictures that differ in emotional salience. Some of these pictures (e.g., that of an amputated human hand) might elicit strong negative reactions in all people, such as feelings of disgust. Dependent variables typically include subjective distress and psychophysiological measures of response before, during, and after viewing these pictures. When using such a paradigm, Gross and colleagues typically observe that providing different instructions on what to do when viewing these pictures can have a dramatic effect on the viewers' subjective and physiological responses.

Specifically, in contrast to suppression, reappraisal more often leads to desirable outcomes. For example, participants reported less distress and arousal when they were asked to reframe emotional pictures in a less distressing way. In contrast, when asked to suppress their emotions while viewing emotional pictures (e.g., by behaving in such a way that nobody would be able to tell how the participant is feeling inside), participants typically experience increased subjective distress and psychophysiological arousal as compared with people who do not attempt to suppress their emotions.

Suppression and reappraisal are the two most widely researched regulation strategies. Gross (1998b) places these strategies at different points in his emotion process model. Figure 5.1 illustrates Gross's process model of emotion regulation. The figure shows the different points of the process that generates the emotional experience (the *emotion generative process*). After a situation is selected, it may be tailored to modify its emotional impact (*situation modification*). Some situations cannot be easily changed (S1x), whereas others allow for some change (S2x–S2z). Furthermore, situations vary in their level of complexity, with some being simple and characterized by only one aspect (a1), whereas others are more complex with many aspects (a1–a5). In a later stage, *attention deployment* may be used to direct the attention focus. During the *cognitive appraisal* stage, the person selects the possible meanings (m1–m3) of a situation. Depending on this selection, emotional response tendencies arise, which are associated with behavioral, experiential, and physiological reactions. Finally, during the *response modulation* stage, the individual may influence the response tendencies after they are activated (e.g., B, B+, B–). The bold arrows indicate an example of one person's strategy.

Results of empirical investigations have so far converged to suggest that antecedent-focused strategies are relatively effective methods of regulating emotion *in the short term*, whereas response-focused strategies tend to be counterproductive (Gross, 1998b; 2002; Gross & John, 2003; Gross & Levenson, 1997).

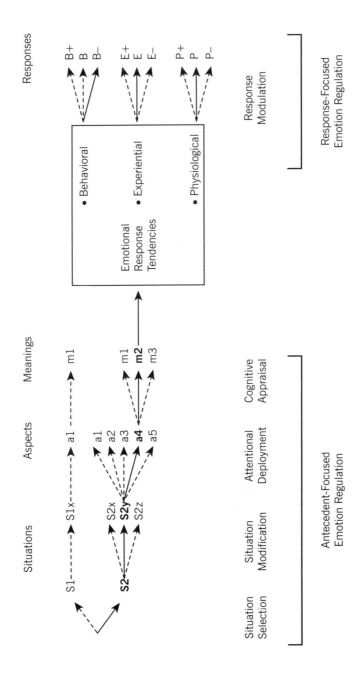

FIGURE 5.1. Gross's process model of emotion regulation. From Gross (1998b). Copyright 1998 by the American Psychological Association. Reprinted by permission.

Effects of Dysregulated Intrapersonal Emotion Regulation

More recently, authors have explored the role of intrapersonal emotion regulation and dysregulation in emotional disorders (for review, see Aldao, Nolen-Hoeksema, & Schweizer, 2010), and especially anxiety disorders (Amstadter, 2008; Cisler, Olatunji, Feldner, & Forsyth, 2010; Hofmann, Sawyer, et al., 2012; Mennin et al., 2005). This literature suggests that individuals who show emotion dysregulation are more prone to developing emotional disorders, such as depression, or are vulnerable to experiencing emotional distress of greater duration and severity than people who do not show these dysregulations. For example, it has been demonstrated that participants with anxiety and mood disorders generally judge their negative affect in response to a distressing film as less acceptable and tend to suppress their emotions to a greater extent than nonanxious participants (Campbell-Sills, Barlow, Brown, & Hofmann, 2006a). Moreover, when instructed to suppress their emotions, individuals with clinical diagnoses of anxiety or depression report higher autonomic arousal than those who are asked to accept their emotions in response to a distressing film during the recovery phase (i.e., patients were asked to simply sit after viewing the film). This finding suggests that suppressing emotional material makes the content more intrusive and persistent than accepting this information (Campbell-Sills, Barlow, Brown, & Hofmann, 2006b).

Similar effects have also been shown in individuals who were asked to undergo a social stress task (Hofmann, Heering, Sawyer, & Asnaani, 2009). In this study, participants were randomly assigned to reappraise, suppress, or accept their anticipatory anxiety prior to an impromptu speech. The instructions to suppress anxiety were associated with greater increase in physiological arousal than the instructions to reappraise and accept. Furthermore, the suppression group reported more subjective anxiety than the reappraisal group. However, the acceptance and suppression groups did not differ in their subjective anxiety response. These findings suggest that both reappraising and accepting anxiety are more effective for moderating physiological arousal than suppressing anxiety but that reappraising is more effective for moderating the subjective feeling of anxiety than attempts to either suppress or accept it. This study showed that cognitive reappraisal of the emotional response to an impromptu speech is more effective at moderating subjective distress and autonomic arousal than attempts to accept or suppress response.

The Suppression Paradox

Studies have shown the paradoxical effects of suppression for regulating pain (Cioffi & Holloway, 1993), craving (Szasz, Szentagotai, & Hofmann, 2012), anger (Szasz, Szentagotai, & Hofmann, 2011), anxiety (Hofmann et al., 2009), embarrassment in nonclinical participants (Harris, 2001), and also in populations with anxiety and mood disorders (Campbell-Sills et al., 2006a, 2006b). Instructions to suppress emotional responses elicited by pictures have also been shown to attenuate the eye-blink startle magnitude (a fear-related physiological response), in comparison with instructions to reappraise or accept (Asnaani, Sawyer, Aderka, & Hofmann, 2013).

The evidence linking emotion suppression to increases in negative affect and physiological arousal can be placed in the larger context of the literature on suppression of other states (e.g., thoughts, pain). Wegner, Schneider, Carter, and White (1987) demonstrated that attempts to suppress thoughts about a white bear paradoxically increased the frequency of such thoughts during a postsuppression period in which participants were free to think about any topic. Subsequent research has established links between this rebound effect as a laboratory phenomenon and clinical disorders. For example, thought suppression has been associated with increased electrodermal responses to emotional thoughts (Wegner & Zanakos, 1994), suggesting that it elevates sympathetic arousal. Evidence also demonstrates that attempts to suppress pain are unproductive (Cioffi & Holloway, 1993). A more detailed discussion of the neurobiology of emotion regulation is presented in Chapter 8.

The apparent paradoxical increase in arousal when trying to suppress an emotion is consistent with studies demonstrating the paradoxical effects of suppressing thoughts or images. In other words, the harder we try not to be bothered by something, the more this something is bothering us. This phenomenon can be observed for virtually any stimuli, including thoughts, images, things in our environment (such as a dripping water faucet or the ticking of a clock), and emotions.

The cognitive self-monitoring that is required to suppress the stimulus leads to the paradoxical effect that the stimulus now becomes intrusive and, due to its intrusiveness, also unpleasant. Moreover, the intrusiveness of the suppressed stimulus tends to linger and continues into the postsuppression period when people are again free to think about any topic (Wegner & Zanakos, 1994). Similarly, attempts to suppress pain are also unproductive (Cioffi & Holloway, 1993).

In Practice: The Paradox of Suppression

Suppressing thoughts, feelings, and behaviors leads to the paradoxical effect that whatever is being suppressed becomes intrusive and takes on a negative valence. The act of suppression requires monitoring, which forces the person to attend to the very issue he or she is trying to avoid. This can be demonstrated with the white bear suppression test (Wegner et al., 1987). In its simplest form, the person receives the following instructions: *(1) Close your eyes and imagine a white bear. Picture it clearly. (2) For 1 minute, think of anything but this white bear. (3) Whenever the bear pops into your mind, lift a finger on your hands to keep track of how many times you thought of the bear. Start now.*

White bears have no specific meaning (and may even be associated with positive feelings). If a thought or image had had personal meaning or was negatively valenced, thought suppression would have been even more challenging and would have evoked negative feelings. For example, the intrusive thought of killing her newborn would make a loving mother very distressed, partly because the image itself is distressing and partly because she might worry that this thought suggests she is crazy or a bad person.

Thus attempts to suppress thoughts or feelings will make the thoughts or feelings more intrusive and disturbing. For this reason, the urge to laugh becomes stronger the harder we try to suppress it. Similarly, the physiological arousal associated with anger becomes stronger the harder we try to suppress our anger. Because of its paradoxical effect, suppression is typically a maladaptive emotion regulation strategy.

Adaptiveness of Emotion Regulation Strategies

Suppression strategies are often maladaptive, whereas reappraisal strategies tend to be more often adaptive, as is discussed in detail in Chapter 6. However, no particular strategy is always adaptive or maladaptive (Bonanno & Burton, 2013). Instead, the question of adaptiveness depends on many factors, including situational demands, context, goal attainment, and the degree to which any strategy is employed. Although the tendency to suppress affect is often cited as an example of a maladaptive strategy, one can think of many situations in which suppression strategies are adaptive, if not essential, in order to adjust to situation demands. For example, it is highly adaptive to suppress anger in some vulnerable interpersonal situations or to suppress the urge to burst out laughing at a funeral of a close relative or friend. On the other hand, suppression strategies can be maladaptive if they lead to unintended, counterproductive effects. For example, attempts to suppress affect increase physiological arousal (Gross, 1998a; Gross & Levenson, 1997). In contrast, taking an accepting stance toward arousing emotions without trying to change or avoid them has been linked to increased persistence in challenging situations and reductions in subjective distress (e.g., Berking, 2010; Hayes, Luoma, Bond, Masuda, & Lillis, 2006; Leahy, Tirch, & Napolitano, 2011).

One possible explanation for the persistent use of ineffective emotion regulation strategies is the acceptability and tolerance of particular emotional experiences (Salovey, Mayer, Goldman, Turvey, & Palfai, 1995). Some people respond to the onset of emotions by appraising them as intolerable and subsequently engage in avoidance, concealment, or other counterproductive response-focused interventions. Recently developed treatments for emotional disorders employ techniques to specifically target such negative judgments of emotions and maladaptive emotional control efforts (e.g., Hayes, Strosahl, & Wilson, 1999; Segal, Williams, & Teasdale, 2002). Mindfulness strategies are often employed with a similar intention.

Emotional Processing

Theorists who examined the role of emotions in psychotherapy adopted an information-processing model (e.g., Greenberg, 2011; Greenberg & Safran, 1987). This model suggests the following therapeutic steps: acknowledging affect, creating meaning, taking responsibility, arousing affect, and modifying affect.

Similarly, Foa and Kozak (1986) adopt an information-processing perspective on emotions. Their treatment model assumes that emotional information is stored in memory in the form of a network. In the case of fear, exposure-based therapy works by integrating new information that is incompatible with existing information about the fear-inducing memory. For example, a child who is afraid of dogs because she believes that all dogs are aggressive will integrate new and incompatible information after interacting with a friendly dog, leading to a change in the existing fear network that incorporates a sense of safety (i.e., "it is safe to interact with dogs"). The same is true for other forms of anxiety-related problems, including fear and avoidance behaviors by traumatized victims. The model assumes that this safety learning is a result of activation of the fear network combined with strong integration of incompatible (i.e, safety-related) information.

A relatively simple strategy to facilitate the processing of emotions (i.e., "working through" the emotional memory and experience) is *structured written disclosure*, also known as *expressive writing* procedure (Pennebaker, 1997). Experiments examining the benefits of expressive writing typically randomize participants to the experimental (expressive writing) condition and a control writing condition. Participants in the experimental condition are asked to write about emotionally upsetting experiences for 15 to 20 minutes a day for 3–4 consecutive days, whereas participants in the control group are asked to write about superficial topics, such as time management. A number of studies have found that expressive writing can positively affect mental and physical health. For example, women with posttraumatic stress disorder reported fewer depressive symptoms after 4 weeks of expressive writing as compared with controls (Sloan & Marx, 2004). Because the expressive writing condition includes instructions to "let go" and exposes people to their emotions by exploring their "deepest thoughts and feelings" about troubling events, it is possible that expressive writing counters the maladaptive cognitive processes, such as rumination and brooding, while exposing individuals to previously avoided feelings. Appendix III gives a clinical example of expressive writing.

Writing about emotions is an effective strategy to facilitate emotional processing. The act of writing and thinking about an emotional event allows us to put some distance between the sources of distress and to gain a more objective perspective of a situation or event.

INTERPERSONAL EMOTION REGULATION

Gross's intrapersonal process model of emotions has been highly influential and has stimulated a great amount of research. However, it is not without weaknesses. First, the model is overly mechanistic, unidimensional, and unidirectional. Although recent formulations of the model (e.g., Gross & John, 2003) consider positive feedback and recursive relationships, the core model identifies a simple input–output relationship between triggers and responses, not unlike a Skinnerian black-box model (despite its emphasis on cognitive factors). Situational factors, such as a context, and expectations are all but ignored in this model. Moreover, some (if not most) emotional experiences, such as fast-acting fear or aggressive responses, cannot be easily explained by this process model, which suggests a slow, multistep process that should require time and deliberations. For example, it is difficult to explain an immediate fear or startle response based on Gross's multistep process model. Finally, and most important, the model does not consider interpersonal processes through which emotions can be regulated (Aldao & Dixon-Gordon, 2014).

Emotion regulation originates in early attachment relationships. An infant's emotional expression becomes the primary means through which attachment figures are made aware of the infant's needs. It has been proposed that what begins as the regulation of basic physiological needs via expressed emotions gradually transforms into emotion regulation (Hofer, 2006). Research on attachment has shown that children utilize the secure base as a means of regulating their emotions as they explore their world (Bowlby, 1973, 1982). When they learn that there is a safe place to turn to when they are distressed, children become more confident that the world is a safe place. This increased confidence is then associated with a reduction of anxiety, allowing infants to move further away from the secure base for extended periods of time (Ainsworth, Blehar, Waters, & Wall, 1978).

Emotion regulation becomes a fundamental aspect of human socialization between the ages of 3 and 6, when social regulation evolves. This is the time when a child learns to respond based on other people's inner states rather than to their outward behaviors and learns to relate the present self to the past self, as well as the future self (Higgins & Pittman, 2008). This learning process depends largely on environmental input in the form of caregivers' verbal and nonverbal reactions to children's emotions, and parents' expression and discussion of emotion (Eisenberg, Spinrad, & Eggum, 2010; Posner & Rothbart, 2000). It develops in the context of parent–child interaction, with both internal and external influences that act on one another over time (Cassidy, 1994; Cole, Martin, & Dennis, 2004; Eisenberg et al., 2010). As executive functioning develops over time, emotion regulation becomes more intentional and effortful (Derryberry & Rothbart, 1997). Therefore, emotion regulation development is closely linked with parental and family influences from early in development, and these influences begin to include the peer context over time (Lunkenheimer, Shields, & Cortina, 2007; Morris, Silk, Steinberg, Myers, & Robinson, 2007).

The development of the affective and cognitive systems underlying emotion regulation continues through adolescence (Silk, Steinberg, & Morris, 2005). For example, the relationship between adolescent emotion and depression is mediated by parents' supportive responses to emotion (Yap, Allen, & Ladouceur, 2008). Research has linked the parents' modeling of processes involved in their own emotion regulation, as well as their responses to children's emotion, to the development of both anxiety and depression (Alloy et al., 2001; Eisenberg et al., 2010; Murray, Creswell, & Cooper, 2009).

Adult attachment relationships mirror the infant–caregiver bond, possibly because of the potential evolutionary advantages of pair bonding (Fraley & Shaver, 2000; Mikulincer & Shaver, 2007). Therefore, adults are likely to experience negative affect when they are socially isolated, whereas social bonding and affiliation are associated with positive affect (Coan, 2010, 2011). This brief discussion of the developmental literature clearly points to the importance of social relationships in emotion regulation. In fact, emotion regulation develops within a social context, incorporating social standards and norms. Throughout development, a person develops strategies to regulate the self and the emotions. Inadequate regulation strategies can lead to emotional distress. Moreover, it has been shown that social support is an important general predictor of psychological health. Social support refers to the psychological and material resources that are needed to reinforce a person's ability to cope with stress (Cohen,

2004). Perceived loneliness and social isolation, an extreme expression of low social support, is a strong predictor of emotional health, especially depression (Cacioppo & Hawkley, 2003; Joiner, 1997). In contrast, social support serves as an important buffer of psychological stress, contributing to resilience in the face of adversities.

The nature of social support can be instrumental (e.g., material things), informational (e.g., guidance to facilitate coping or problem solving), and emotional (e.g., empathy). Perceived social support appears to be more important than received (enacted) social support for emotional health (Haber, Cohen, Lucas, & Baltes, 2007; Lakey, Orehek, Hain, & Van Vleet, 2010), such as depression (e.g., Brown & Harris, 1978; George, Blazer, Hughes & Fowler, 1989; Stice, Ragan, & Randall, 2004; Travis, Lyness, Shields, King, & Cox, 2004). However, the mechanism through which social support affects emotional well-being is not well understood. It has been proposed that interpersonal emotion regulation might serve as a proximal mechanism through which social support affects emotional well-being (Marroquín, 2011).

A recently proposed framework of interpersonal emotion regulation (Hofmann, 2014; Zaki & Williams, 2013) distinguishes *intrinsic* versus *extrinsic* and *response-independent* versus *response-dependent* interpersonal emotion regulation strategies. *Intrinsic interpersonal regulation* refers to the process by which one person's emotions are regulated by recruiting the help of other people. In contrast, *extrinsic emotion regulation* is the process by which one person regulates another person's emotions. These processes can be response-dependent or response-independent. They are response-dependent if the processes rely on a particular response by another person, and they are response-independent if they do not require that the interaction partner respond in any particular way (or if the partner may not be able to do so).

In the case of *intrinsic* interpersonal emotion regulation, a person wants to regulate his or her emotion through the help of another person. An example may be Kathleen, a woman with panic disorder and agoraphobia who is afraid of going to a mall alone. Kathleen is able to do this with either her husband or a doctor friend (Dr. Smith) by her side. By asking her husband or Dr. Smith to accompany her to the mall, Kathleen is able to regulate (i.e., reduce) her anxiety. Kathleen's anxiety is regulated through slightly different interpersonal factors by her husband and Dr. Smith.

Kathleen's motives to have her husband and Dr. Smith by her side are slightly different. Simply feeling the presence of her loving husband makes Kathleen feel more at ease, even if he should be unable to effectively respond in any particular way if she experiences a medical emergency ("you will stand by me"). Similarly, Kathleen's husband might suggest to Kathleen that he accompany her to the mall for the same reason ("feel my love"). The former is an example of intrinsic response-independent interpersonal emotion regulation, and the latter is an example of extrinsic response-dependent interpersonal emotion regulation.

In contrast to her husband, Kathleen's friend, Dr. Smith, has medical training and could effectively intervene in case Kathleen experiences a medical emergency, which is an example of a *response-dependent emotion regulation*. Depending on whether the regulation is motivated by Kathleen ("you will rescue me") or Dr. Smith ("I need to make you feel better"), we can again distinguish between *intrinsic* and *extrinsic response-dependent emotion regulation*. Accordingly, these orthogonal processes create a 2 × 2 matrix: extrinsic versus intrinsic processes that are either response-dependent or response-independent (Figure 5.2).

Just as intrapersonal strategies can be maladaptive or adaptive in regulating emotions, interpersonal strategies as well can be adaptive (if they serve as a buffer of emotion stress) or maladaptive (if they contribute to the maintenance of the problem). The presence of a safety person is an example of a maladaptive emotion regulation strategy. A safety person provides Kathleen a sense of security, leading to a reduction in the level of her fear typically associated with entering a mall and thereby acting as an emotion regulation strategy. Clinically, it is considered a maladaptive strategy because the presence of the safety person in effect leads to the maintenance of Kathleen's irrational fear of entering a mall. Frequent or habitual use of interpersonal emotion regulation strategies can conceivably reduce a patient's sense of control of his or her own emotion experience. Therefore, interpersonal emotion regulation can become maladaptive if a patient becomes dependent on specific individuals or social groups in order to regulate his or her own affect.

	Classes of regulation	
	Intrinsic	**Extrinsic**
Response-independent	"You will stand by me." Kathleen asks her husband to accompany her to the mall.	"Feel my love." Kathleen's husband suggests to Kathleen that he accompany her to the mall.
Response-dependent	"You will rescue me." Dr. Smith agrees to Kathleen's request to accompany her to the mall so that Dr. Smith can intervene in case of an emergency.	"I need to make you feel better." Dr. Smith suggests to Kathleen that she accompany Kathleen to the mall in case of an emergency.

(Left margin label spanning rows: **Mechanisms**)

FIGURE 5.2. Examples of interpersonal emotion regulation strategies. Kathleen is suffering from panic disorder and agoraphobia and is afraid of going to the mall.

Extending emotion regulation to include interpersonal processes offers an interesting transdiagnostic perspective of emotional disorders. Furthermore, it considers the broader (social) context of an individual's behavior and emotional experience. Despite these advantages, an interpersonal model of emotion regulation shows a number of weaknesses. First, there are no instruments available yet to measure interpersonal emotion regulation strategies. Therefore, the direct empirical evidence for the impact of these strategies on emotional distress is relatively weak. Any assessment instrument will need to consider the influence of the cultural context because interpersonal emotion regulation strategies are directly related to social standards and expectations. Finally, it remains unknown how interpersonal and intrapersonal emotion regulation strategies interact, and the relative importance of these groups of strategies combined are unexplored.

Interpersonal Emotion Regulation in Anxiety Disorders

Whenever individuals are in close relationships, emotion regulation is probably not limited to intrapersonal regulation strategies but will also include interpersonal strategies. For those with chronic disorders, these strategies are likely to be maladaptive, contributing to the maintenance of the disorders. In the case of anxiety disorders, avoidance behaviors are some of the primary maintenance factors (e.g., Barlow, 2002; Foa & Kozak, 1986; Solomon & Wynne, 1953). The presence of safety persons constitutes an example of such an avoidance strategy. Framed in the interpersonal emotion regulation model, safety people contribute to the maintenance of an anxiety disorder by serving as maladaptive response-dependent and response-independent intrinsic interpersonal emotion regulation strategies.

Whether intentionally or not, the safety person reduces the patient's distress by creating a sense of safety. Through repeated and prolonged exposure to threat in the absence of safety signals (e.g., safety persons) and avoidance behaviors, the individual is able to reevaluate the perceived danger of a situation, leading to changes in harm expectancy and anxious apprehension (e.g., Hofmann, 2008). These changes are more likely to occur if internal fear cues and other significant contexts are systematically produced (e.g., Bouton, Mineka, & Barlow, 2001) and if the outcome of the feared situation is unexpectedly positive because it forces the person to reevaluate the actual threat of the situation.

The process of extinction learning is best understood as new learning (e.g., the acquisition of a sense of safety in a social situation) rather than weakening of a previously learned fear association. The interpersonal model of emotion regulation provides an additional theoretical framework within which to understand the interpersonal and social context that contributes to the maintenance of anxiety. Educating the patient's partner about his or her role in this process might further strengthen the efficacy of the exposure procedures. Following is a dialogue among Kathleen, a patient with panic disorder and agoraphobia, Mike, her husband, and the therapist.

In Practice: The Safety Person

THERAPIST: It is nice to finally meet you, Mike. I heard a lot of good things about you from Kathleen.

MIKE: It's nice meeting you, too.

THERAPIST: Did Kathleen mention to you why I thought we should have a session together?

MIKE: Yes. She said that you want to talk to me about how I can help her with her panic problem.

THERAPIST: That's right. As you know, Kathleen has been working hard between our sessions with some of the exposures, and you have been helping her quite a bit.

MIKE: That's right. We even took a longer route to get to your office to drive over the Zakim Bridge twice.

THERAPIST: That's terrific. How did it go, Kathleen?

KATHLEEN: I think it went pretty well. I was still very nervous, but I was able to do it. I am just really glad that Mike was sitting next to me.

THERAPIST: Do you think you could have done it without having Mike in the car?

KATHLEEN: I am not sure; maybe. It really helps me a lot when Mike is there.

THERAPIST: It's really terrific that you feel so comfortable around Mike. You obviously have a very supportive relationship, and this is clearly very special. You obviously care for each other a lot. Mike's presence clearly makes the exposures easier for you. We have seen this also with a number of other exercises from the previous weeks. Can you see anything wrong with this?

KATHLEEN: You mean that Mike is so supportive?

THERAPIST: No, I don't think that there is anything wrong with Mike being a generally supportive husband. This is really wonderful. What I mean is: Do you think that there is a problem with having Mike there during the exposures? What is the difference between having Mike there versus doing the exposures alone? Which is more difficult?

KATHLEEN: Oh, clearly, when I have to do it alone.

THERAPIST: Why?

KATHLEEN: Because Mike makes me feel better.

THERAPIST: Mike, what do you think?

MIKE: I will do whatever I can do to beat that thing.

THERAPIST: Right, and that's the reason why I asked to you to join today's session. Panic is a horrible experience. It is very debilitating, and I completely understand why you want to accompany Kathleen to her exposures, and I completely understand why Kathleen wants to have you there during the exposures. It makes sense in the short term because the exposures are more bearable. However, it also brings up a serious problem for the long term. Mike's presence makes the exposures for Kathleen easier, because Mike has become something that we call a *safety person*. The term *safety person* sounds good, but it is really a big problem. Having a *safety person* there during an exposure is a specific form of avoidance. You don't avoid the situation per se, but you are avoiding confronting your anxiety on your own, and you will continue to feel fearful of the same situation unless you can face your fear without any avoidance strategies. Kathleen, why don't you explain to Mike how avoidance maintains anxiety? I would like Mike to become my cotherapist to help out with the exposures between sessions, and I think we need to update him about what we were discussing.

Interpersonal Emotion Regulation in Mood Disorders

Although there is a relatively large literature examining the associations between depression and marital interaction, the findings are ambiguous and contradictory (for a review, see Rehman, Gollan, & Mortimer, 2008). Marital distress and depression are closely associated and interrelated (e.g., Fincham, Beach, Harold, & Osborne, 1997). The majority of studies in this area examine communication within a conflict or problem-solving paradigm. These studies suggest that marital communication in a relationship in which one spouse is depressed is characterized by more frequent negative communication and less frequent positive communication (Johnson & Jacob, 1997; Rehman et al., 2008). Therefore, most intervention studies have attempted to improve communication patterns using behavioral principles. However, these studies have revealed disappointing results (e.g., Rehman et al., 2008).

Different intervention targets emerge when adopting the interpersonal emotion regulation view. For example, it has been shown that helping behaviors of husbands were viewed less positively by wives who showed depressive symptoms (Pasch, Bradbury, & Davila, 1997). Similarly, maladaptive communication was not consistently associated with depression but depended on the wife's emotional state: Wives communicated more negatively with husbands in a problem-solving task only when they reported depressive symptoms and underwent a negative mood induction (Rehman, Ginting, Karimiha, & Goodnight, 2010). In other words, the wife's emotional state moderated the relationship between marital conflict and depression. Therefore, communication trainings are unlikely to succeed unless the functional relationship between the partner's behaviors and the patient's emotions is being addressed (i.e., How does the partner contribute to the patient's maladaptive emotion regulation strategies?). For example, the husband might employ extrinsic interpersonal emotion regulation toward his wife in order to deal with his own frustration at work. Kathleen's husband might reinforce her dependency on him to compensate for his own insecurity and fear that she might leave him if she becomes more independent. Providing communication and problem-solving training without considering such interpersonal emotion regulation processes might even accentuate the patient's presenting problem. The case of Kathleen illustrates these processes and mechanisms of interpersonal emotion regulation.

Summary of Clinically Relevant Points

- Emotion regulation involves maintaining, enhancing, and inhibiting emotions. By regulating emotions, we can influence the valence, intensity, and temporal features of an emotion. Emotions are not only modified through self-regulation strategies, but they can also be regulated by others. Emotion regulation involves a function (i.e., emotions are regulated for a reason and are directed toward a goal).

- Intrapersonal emotion regulation can be broadly distinguished into *response-focused* and *antecedent-focused* strategies, depending on the timing during the emotion-generative process. Antecedent-focused emotion regulation strategies occur before the emotional response has been fully activated and include situation modification, attention deployment, and cognitive reframing of a situation. In contrast, response-focused emotion regulation strategies entail attempts to alter the expression or experience of emotions after response tendencies have been initiated, such as suppression and other experiential avoidance strategies.

- Emotion regulation strategies per se are neither good nor bad. Rather, effectiveness depends on the adaptiveness of an emotion regulation strategy to the particular situational demand and goal achievement.

- Emotion regulation not only involves intrapersonal but also interpersonal processes. These interpersonal processes can result in a maladaptive equilibrium, leading to the maintenance of emotional disorders.

CHAPTER SIX

◆

Appraisal and Reappraisal

Although emotions appear to happen automatically, we do have control over them—at least to some extent. Reappraisal is, generally speaking, the most effective (i.e., generally most adaptive) intrapersonal emotion regulation strategy. Reappraising emotion-eliciting stimuli is closely linked to the core processes of cognitive therapy, as described and introduced into modern psychotherapy by Beck (1979) and Ellis (1962). The emotional response to an event depends on its interpretation, and the interpretation of an event is influenced by a number of factors, including one's schemas, the context, past experiences, and so forth. These factors provide the filter that determines which interpretation (and thus which emotional reaction) is more likely. A recent environmental experience in Boston might illustrate this point. A few days before I wrote this paragraph, Virginia and the District of Columbia experienced a sizeable earthquake of the magnitude of 5.3, sending waves far across the northeast, even to Boston and New York. The tremors in Boston were minor, causing no damages, but they lasted 20 seconds and were clearly noticeable.

Depending on the context, the minor earthquake was interpreted in many different ways by different people. One person from my gym thought the slight movement of the ground he felt suggested a physical crisis, possibly a stroke or heart attack. A friend attributed it to the subway construction project close to her building. Both of these initial interpretations turned out to be inaccurate and were replaced with the accurate interpretation once more information became available. Context, past experience, and prior knowledge contributed to these initially inaccurate interpretations of the event (e.g., rigorous exercise can lead to a stroke that may be associated with odd perceptions and movement problems; construction work in the subway system can cause buildings to shake). Moreover, these different interpretations led to different emotional responses. The person at the gym was scared, my friend annoyed.

THE COGNITIVE-BEHAVIORAL APPROACH

The cognitive-behavioral approach to treating emotional disorders is based on the assumption that our behavioral and emotional responses are determined by our appraisal of situations and events rather than the situations and events themselves. In other words, we are only anxious, angry, or sad if we think we have reason to be anxious, angry, or sad. Thus it is not the situation per se but, rather, our perceptions, expectations, and interpretations (i.e., the cognitive appraisal) of events that trigger the emotions. This might be best explained by the following example provided by Beck (1979):

> A housewife hears a door slam. Several hypotheses occur to her: "It may be Sally returning from school." "It might be a burglar." "It might be the wind that blew the door shut." The favored hypothesis should depend on her taking into account all the relevant circumstances. The logical process of hypothesis testing may be disrupted, however, by the housewife's psychological set. If her thinking is dominated by the concept of danger, she might jump to the conclusion that it is a burglar. She makes an arbitrary inference. Although such an inference is not necessarily incorrect, it is based primarily on internal cognitive processes rather than actual information. If she then runs and hides, she postpones or forfeits the opportunity to disprove (or confirm) the hypothesis. (pp. 234–235)

In short, the same initial event (hearing the slamming of the door) can elicit very different emotion responses, depending on how one interprets the situational context. The slamming of the door itself does not elicit any emotions one way or the other. However, if the woman assumed that the door slam suggested there was a burglar in the house, she would likely have experienced fear because, in this case, the door slam would have signaled potential danger. The likelihood for this interpretation would be further increased if she was primed after watching a horror movie or reading about burglaries in the paper. She would also be more likely to come to this conclusion if her core belief (also known as a *schema*) was that the world is dangerous place. Her behavior, of course, would be very different if she thought the event had no significant meaning or if the door slamming signaled for her a joyful or neutral event (e.g., the return of her husband).

In the context of cognitive therapy, the assumptions about events and situations are often referred to as *automatic thoughts,* because these thoughts arise spontaneously, without much prior reflection or reasoning (e.g., Beck, 1979). These thoughts are based on general, overarching core beliefs, or *schemas*, that the person has about him- or herself, the world, and the future. These core beliefs or schemas determine how a person may interpret a specific situation and thereby determine the range and likelihood of specific automatic thoughts. These specific automatic thoughts contribute to the person's maladaptive cognitive appraisal of the situation or event, leading to an emotional response. The word *maladaptive* here suggests that the appraisal does not serve an adaptive function. *Adaptive* in this context refers to the ability to adapt to life's challenges, generally speaking.

Other cognitions are expressed in the form of *self-statements,* because they are statements that the person tells him- or herself in order to interpret the events in the external world (Ellis, 1962). In his A-B-C model, Ellis illustrates the relationship between these events, cognitions, and emotional responses. In this model, A stands for the antecedent event (the door slam), B stands for belief ("It must be a burglar"), and C stands for consequence (fear). If the thought occurs so quickly and automatically that the person reacts almost reflexively to the activating event, without critical reflection, B can also stand for *blank*. Unless the cognition is in the center of the person's awareness, it can be difficult to identify it. This is the reason that Beck refers to it as an *automatic* thought. Therefore, a cognitive therapist encourages the patient to relate a specific scenario or circumstance that preceded a low mood, for example. The therapist and patient carefully observe the sequence of events and the patient's response to them, identify any automatic thoughts that may be behind her or his response, and explore the underlying belief system supporting those automatic thoughts.

Despite some minor differences between the Ellis and Beck models, both stress the idea that distorted cognitions are at the center of psychological problems. These cognitions are considered distorted because they are misperceptions and misinterpretations of situations and events, typically do not reflect reality, are maladaptive, and lead to emotional distress, behavior problems, and unhelpful physiological arousal. The specific patterns of physiological symptoms, emotional distress, and dysfunctional behaviors that result from this process are interpreted as syndromes of mental disorders. A general reappraisal model, based on Beck's (1979) and Ellis's (1962) conceptualizations, is presented in Figure 6.1.

This model illustrates that maladaptive trait cognitions, which are often general beliefs (schemas), can lead to maladaptive specific state cognitions. These maladaptive state cognitions can be automatic when attention is allocated to certain triggers, such as situations, events, sensations, or even other thoughts. The processes that lead to the allocation of attention to these stimuli can happen on a subconscious level and often show a high degree of automaticity. For example, people with panic disorder are often hypervigilant to subtle bodily changes and frequently scan their bodies subconsciously for possible abnormalities. Once the person is consciously aware of the focus of his or her attention, the triggers are interpreted and evaluated. This appraisal then leads to a subjective experience, physiological symptoms, and a behavioral response associated with the emotion. For example, most people are not consciously aware of the heart palpitations induced by the caffeine from a strong cup of coffee. In contrast, the patient with panic disorder who just had a strong cup of coffee might interpret heart palpitations as a sign of an impending heart attack rather than to an innocuous response to coffee. As

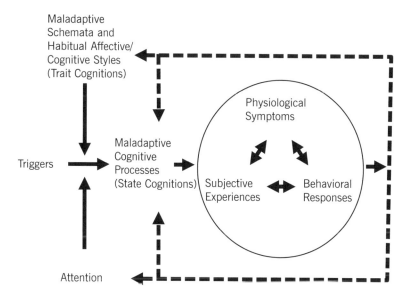

FIGURE 6.1. General cognitive-behavioral model. From Hofmann (2011). Copyright 2012 by Wiley & Sons. Adapted by permission.

another example, a person who believes the statement "I am socially incompetent" is more likely to interpret an event (e.g., an audience member yawning when the person is giving a presentation) in a way that is consistent with that belief: "She is yawning because I have no social skills." This interpretation of the situation then leads to subjective experience (fear and embarrassment), physiological symptoms (heart racing), and behavioral responses (stuttering). These symptoms and responses can distract from the actual task performance, further supporting the maladaptive cognitive appraisal of the situation and the schema the person holds of being incompetent, establishing a positive feedback loop and vicious cycle.

Interestingly, this positive feedback loop can also be reinforced by emotional reasoning, which is a maladaptive cognitive process that uses one's emotional experience as evidence for the validity of a thought (Bem, 1967; Festinger & Carlsmith, 1959; Schachter & Singer, 1962). For example, a person who is afraid of dogs may believe the fear of dogs is evidence for the notion that dogs must be dangerous. Emotional reasoning establishes a positive feedback loop by turning a consequence of a thought (e.g., fear of dogs) into an antecedent of the same thought (e.g., dogs are dangerous). This kind of positive feedback loop can be seen in many emotional disorders.

Separating the emotional response into subjective experience, physiology, and behavior may seem artificial, and some schools of psychology believe that it is unnecessary to make such a division. For example, proponents of behavior analysis may argue that every response to an event or a situation is a behavioral response and thus that it is not useful to assume that cognitive appraisal precedes the response or that subjective and physiological responses are distinct from overt behavioral responses. However, as shown throughout this book, there is sufficient evidence to support the cognitive-behavioral model. Moreover, it is a clinically useful model when formulating specific intervention strategies.

The three components, subjective experience, physiology, and behavior, form a system together but can be targeted separately. In the case of anxiety, the behavioral component often takes the form of avoidance strategies with the goal of improving or eliminating the unpleasant state the person experiences. Other avoidance strategies can be experiential in nature. For example, the person might avoid the subjective experience or physiological sensations of an emotional response rather than the situation per se. However, avoidance strategies are maladaptive and lead to the maintenance of the problem because they do not allow the system to change by considering any disconfirming evidence. Moreover, emotional reasoning strengthens the positive feedback loop, further stabilizing the system. At the core of this system, however, are maladaptive thoughts. These thoughts serve as triggers and mediate the response to events in our environment.

MALADAPTIVE APPRAISAL

Human reasoning consists of two separate cognitive systems. System 1 is intuitive, quick, low-effort, and association-based, whereas System 2 is deliberate, slow, effortful, and logical (Kahneman, 2011). Both cognitive systems can be maladaptive and can instigate or heighten emotional distress. Cognitive-behavioral therapy (CBT) strategies address both systems by encouraging the person to become a rational and critical thinker and scientist, identifying and modifying maladaptive beliefs.

As noted earlier, the word *maladaptive* suggests that the beliefs do not serve an adaptive function, whereas *adaptive* beliefs are helpful in adapting to life's challenges, generally speaking. Life is precious and can be short, and unexpected, undesirable, and even traumatic things are part of life. Relationships can end and one might lose his or her job or develop a serious chronic disease. None of these tragedies happen often, fortunately, but it is unlikely that any person lives a life free from tragedies. To make things worse, no matter how happy we are at any given moment, everything is eventually coming to an end; sooner or later we, our loved ones, and the rest of the human race will cease to exist.

Clearly, there are plenty of reasons to be depressed. However, the majority of people encountering adverse events are not depressed, despite these challenges and the nature of life itself. One crucial difference between those who remain emotionally healthy, happy, and resilient and those who become depressed and emotionally distressed is the perspective they take toward these events, the future, and life in general. People who remain emotionally healthy in the presence of adversities often show a positive bias toward events and are optimistic about the future. They are also more likely to attribute positive events to themselves and attribute negative events to other causes (Menzulis, Abramson, Hyde, & Hankin, 2004). This *self-serving attributional bias* is often missing or deficient in people who are emotionally distressed. Individuals with depression often tend to attribute negative events to internal (something about the self), stable (enduring), and global (general) causes (e.g., lack of ability, personality flaws). Adopting such an attributional style leads one to conclude that negative events are likely to recur in the future throughout a wide variety of domains, leading to widespread hopelessness (Abramson & Seligman, 1978).

In addition to having a self-serving attributional bias, healthy people show a bias that emphasizes the positive aspects of a situation and deemphasizes the negative attributes, while experiencing an illusion of control over the future (Alloy & Clements, 1992). It could be argued that depression, for example, is partly the result of a breakdown of positive cognitive biases, perhaps resulting in a more realistic but maladaptive assessment of the uncontrollable and unpredictable nature of events. This idea has also been referred to as *depressive realism* (Alloy & Clements, 1992; Mischel, 1979; Moore & Fresco, 2012) and is consistent with the notion that, in contrast to people with depression, healthy people show a remarkable degree of resiliency when confronted with adversities. People will often use their current state as the basis to predict how they might feel in the future if a particular event happens to them (Gilbert & Wilson, 2007). Because we tend to be constrained by the present moment, we tend to be inaccurate when it comes to such affective forecasting. In other words, we tend to overestimate how happy we will be if we win the lottery, but we also overestimate how sad we will be if our spouse dies. In people with depression, affective forecasting appears to be biased in such a way that they cannot imagine liking future events (MacLeod & Cropley, 1996).

Maladaptive cognitions are often expressed in the form of situation-specific thoughts (Burns, 1980). Although maladaptive cognitions are disorder-specific, there are a number of commonalities of cognitions shared by emotional disorders. Many maladaptive cognitions in emotional disorders are associated with perceptions of threat to self or loss. In the case of anxiety disorders, this sense of danger may involve either physical (e.g., having a heart attack) or psychological (e.g., anxiety focused on embarrassment) threat. In the case of depression, the maladaptive cognitions often revolve around loss and self-worth. In addition, these cognitions tend to focus upon a sense of uncontrollability over the situation or the symptoms of anxiety. Another hallmark of anxious cognitions is that they tend to be automatic or habitual, such that conjuring up such thoughts requires little effort. They occur instantaneously and sometimes in response to subtle cues.

Common Maladaptive Cognitions

There are all kinds of maladaptive cognitions, also known as thinking errors. The following categories of these cognitions arise especially frequently.

- *Black-and-white thinking.* People who engage in this thinking style divide reality into two discrete categories that are either *good* (white) or *bad* (black). An example might be the person who thinks that even a minor stumble during a professional presentation means that the performance was a complete disaster.

- *Personalization.* Undesirable events can happen to everybody. However, some people take them personally and see themselves solely responsible for these events, although they are not. For example, a public speaker who sees a person in the audience yawning might conclude that this means that he or she is a boring speaker.

- *Focusing on the negatives.* Any given situation usually contains both positive and negative aspects. For a person with a bias to focus on negative aspects of a situation, those aspects then become the center of attention. For example, the speaker who noticed the yawn in the audience might then look for further evidence to support his or her perception that people are bored.

- *Disqualifying the positives.* The person with such a negative bias not only focuses on the negative aspects but also ignores or dismisses any positive aspects. Therefore, the speaker who believes that his or her speech is boring is likely to ignore the other audience members who attentively listen to the speech.

- *Jumping to conclusions.* The conclusion "I am boring" after seeing somebody yawn in the audience is a leap that is not well justified. Yet the speaker might be convinced that this is an already established fact.

- *Overgeneralization.* The label "I am boring" or "I am a boring speaker" suggests that all future presentations will be boring. Thus a negative event turns into a never-ending pattern.

- *Catastrophizing.* Catastrophizing occurs when a person blows things out of proportion. For example, the speaker who sees an audience member yawn not only concludes that he or she is a boring person but that this may also mean that his or her career is over, and that he or she will get fired and will never find a job again.

- *Probability overestimation.* The person believes that an unlikely event is likely to happen. For example, plane crashes can and do happen. However, the likelihood of dying in a plane crash is very low, given the number of planes that depart and land safely each day.

• *Emotional reasoning.* Emotional reasoning happens when a person interprets an emotional response to a thought as evidence for the validity of this thought. For example, worrying about losing one's job causes distress. At the same time, a person who engages in emotional reasoning concludes that the distress experienced during the worrying is a sign that there is good reason to worry (i.e., "I must have good reason to worry about X because I am feeling distress when I am thinking about X").

This is not an exhaustive list, and the categories greatly overlap. However, labeling and categorizing distressing thoughts are often important steps toward distancing oneself from these thoughts and obtaining a more rational perspective of a situation rather than a biased perspective leading to maladaptive emotional responses.

REAPPRAISAL TECHNIQUES

In CBT, a thought is treated not as factual or accurate but as one of many hypotheses. After all, it is usually possible to interpret a situation in a number of different ways. Reappraisal can transform a maladaptive interpretation of a situation or event into an adaptive interpretation of the same situation or event. Often maladaptive interpretations are flawed perceptions. But this is not necessarily so; a flawed thought can be adaptive and an accurate thought can be maladaptive. As described earlier, there is good reason to be depressed given the many adversities that can and do happen (and given the cruel fact that all will eventually come to an end). The critical difference between people with and without depression lies in the prominence of maladaptive, not inaccurate, beliefs. In fact, some research suggests that depressed people have a more accurate view of the world, which is known as depressive realism (Moore & Fresco, 2012). For the majority of cases, however, maladaptive beliefs are also inaccurate beliefs.

The first step in reappraisal requires the person to entertain the idea that the initial assumption might be incorrect. This, in turn, requires some degree of cognitive flexibility and the capacity to shift one's perspective. It also requires the willingness to accept that the initial interpretation did not match the truth (and that there may even be more than one truth).

All of these deliberations are relatively complex; they include self-awareness, as well as metacognitive awareness—the awareness of one's thoughts and beliefs about one's thoughts. This level of awareness can be achieved in a patient by encouraging her or him to adopt a neutral observer role instead of being a continuous actor and reactor to situational triggers. In the next step, the patient gathers evidence for and against a particular interpretation of the situation or stimuli. This puts the thought "on trial" and, as in a scientific test, the hypothesis is either refuted or supported by the evidence.

It is not an easy task to identify, challenge, and modify maladaptive thoughts. In therapy, the therapist often asks guiding questions to encourage the patient to explore alternative ways of interpretation. This process often requires careful self-exploration by the patient and guided questioning (or guided discovery) by the therapist (which has been referred to as a Socratic questioning style in Beckian CBT). Like any bad habit, the way we interpret things tends to be resistant to change. The first step toward change is to realize that there are many different ways an event can be interpreted. In order to interpret an event, we need to formulate hypotheses, which ultimately determine our emotional response to the event. The following example illustrates Socratic questioning in a therapy session with a patient who has panic disorder and agoraphobia.

In Practice: Socratic Questioning

THERAPIST: Why do you not like crowded malls?

KATHLEEN: Because they make me very uncomfortable. When I step into a mall, I feel like I am having an anxiety attack.

THERAPIST: What usually happens when you are having anxiety attacks?

KATHLEEN: I get very frightened.

THERAPIST: Why are you getting afraid?

KATHLEEN: I don't know. I sometimes think that there is something wrong with me . . . that I have a heart attack or something like that.

THERAPIST: Is your heart pounding really fast?

KATHLEEN: Yes, it is racing.

THERAPIST: Why do you think this means there is something wrong with your heart?

KATHLEEN: Well, because this can signal a heart attack.

THERAPIST: How many heart attacks have you had?

KATHLEEN: None, my doctor says that everything looks OK.

THERAPIST: So then how do you know that those are symptoms of a heart attack?

KATHLEEN: I don't, but I am afraid that they might be.

THERAPIST: So you *think* these symptoms are related to a heart attack, but you are not sure. How high would you rate the probability that these symptoms are related to a heart attack on a scale from 0—not likely—to 100—very likely?

KATHLEEN: Maybe 40%.

THERAPIST: This means there is a 40% chance that you are having a heart attack when you experience the symptoms of palpitations, chest pain, and breathlessness in the mall.

KATHLEEN: Yes.

THERAPIST: So out of ten visits to the mall, on four occasions you will have experienced a heart attack. Is this correct?

KATHLEEN: No, this sounds too high.

In this example, the therapist began challenging Kathleen's maladaptive thought that anxiety attacks, and especially heart palpitations experienced in the mall, are signs of a heart attack. It is certainly not impossible to experience a heart attack in a crowded place, including a mall. However, Kathleen is a young healthy woman with no cardiovascular disease. Therefore, the likelihood that she will experience a heart attack in a mall is low. Therefore, this thought (that there is a 40% chance her anxious feelings in a mall indicate a heart attack) is an example of a probability overestimation.

In order to put this thought to the test, Kathleen will need to conduct a number of tests to examine the validity of her beliefs. For example, she might confront a crowded mall, possibly even after some strenuous physical exercises to induce heart palpitations. This will provide an opportunity to test her prediction that she will experience a heart attack. Such "field experiments" are essential to examine the validity of specific assumptions. These assumptions are maladaptive because they are catastrophic misinterpretations of the rush of physical sensations experienced during a panic attack ("I'm having a heart attack," "I'm losing my mind," "I'm going to lose control") and thus lead to an increase in her anxiety and ultimately her inability to go to the mall. If Kathleen was able to attribute her panic symptoms to some more innocuous cause, it would be less likely that clinical levels of anxiety would result.

MALADAPTIVE SCHEMAS

Schemas are general, overarching beliefs that give rise to specific automatic thoughts in a given situation. These schemas develop early on, often during childhood and adolescence. Sometimes they take the form of *maladaptive schemas*, which are broad, pervasive beliefs comprising skewed emotions, cognitions, bodily sensations, and memories regarding oneself and one's relationships with others (Young, Klosko, & Weishaar, 2003). These maladaptive schemas underlie long-standing characterological problems and are viewed as general vulnerability factors for a broad range of psychiatric disorders.

Maladaptive schemas occur when temperament interacts with early adverse relational experiences, leading the person to feel that his or her psychological core needs (e.g., secure attachment, autonomy, freedom to express valid needs and emotions, realistic limits) are not met (Young et al., 2003). When a schema is triggered later, the person responds with a maladaptive coping style (e.g., overcompensation, avoidance, surrender) that he or she learned as a way to cope with these adverse experiences and that in fact perpetuates the schema. According to Young et al. (2003), 15 maladaptive schemas can develop. These are:

- Abandonment/instability (the perceived instability or unreliability of significant others for emotional support and connection).
- Mistrust/abuse (expectation that others will abuse, humiliate, manipulate, hurt, or intentionally take advantage of oneself).

- Emotional deprivation (expectation that one's needs for empathy, protection, and nurturance will not be met by others).
- Defectiveness/shame (belief that one is flawed, defective, and unlovable to significant others).
- Social isolation (feeling that one is isolated from the world, different from others, and is not part of a peer group or community).
- Dependence (belief that one is incapable of handling day-to-day responsibilities independently and competently).
- Vulnerability to harm (exaggerated fear that an imminent and unpreventable catastrophe will strike at any moment, such as a natural, financial, medical, or relationship crisis).
- Enmeshment (excessive emotional overinvolvement and closeness with significant others at the expense of one's individuation).
- Failure (belief that, compared with peers, one is fundamentally inadequate in areas of achievement).
- Entitlement (belief that one should be able to do what one wants to do regardless of what is considered reasonable to others or realistic).
- Insufficient self-control (difficulty in exercising sufficient self-control and frustration in achieving one's goals and restraining expression of impulses and feelings).
- Subjugation (belief that one has to surrender control to others to avoid negative consequences).
- Self-sacrifice (focus on meeting the needs of others at the expense of one's own).
- Emotional inhibition (belief that one must inhibit spontaneous emotions and actions to avoid disapproval by others or feelings of shame).
- Unrelenting standards (belief that one must strive to meet very high standards of performance and behaviors).

As part of CBT, and especially in later sessions, therapists often explore and target such maladaptive schemas. An assessment of Kathleen's schemas (see pp. 113–114) suggests that her fear of panic attacks in malls and other situations is associated with the schemas *abandonment/instability* and *vulnerability to harm*.

A detailed description of the techniques for identifying and targeting maladaptive schemas is given in Young et al. (2003). Although these techniques are part of CBT, there is also some overlap to object relations and gestalt therapy. For example, some of the techniques for targeting these schemas instruct the patient to create images of significant people (e.g., father, mother), to conduct dialogues with the individuals in these images, and to link emotions from childhood images with present life circumstances. The therapeutic relationship creates a context in which to trigger schemas safely and to test their validity by using evidence from all periods of the patient's life. Schemas can also be modified when the therapist provides limited parenting by helping to fulfill the patient's needs that were not adequately met.

REAPPRAISAL AND EMOTIONS

A large body of research points to the efficacy of CBT for a wide range of mental disorders. A recent review of meta-analyses examining the efficacy of CBT identified no fewer than 269 meta-analytic studies (Hofmann, Asnaani, Vonk, Sawyer, & Fang, 2012). The meta-analyses examined CBT for substance use disorder, schizophrenia and other psychotic disorders, depression and dysthymia, bipolar disorder, anxiety disorders, somatoform disorders, eating disorders, insomnia, personality disorders, anger and aggression, criminal behaviors, general stress, distress due to general medical conditions, chronic pain and fatigue, and distress related to pregnancy complications and female hormonal conditions. Additional meta-analytic reviews examined the efficacy of CBT for various problems in children and elderly adults. The strongest support for CBT exists for anxiety disorders, somatoform disorders, bulimia, anger control problems, and general stress.

These studies also support the efficacy of reappraisal strategies on emotional and behavioral problems, because reappraisal is a core element of CBT. However, modern CBT protocols are not solely based on reappraisal (Hofmann, Asmundson, & Beck, 2013), but include many other strategies (Hofmann, 2011). The same is true for virtually any psychosocial intervention. This makes it difficult to compare the various interventions directly with each other, let alone to identify the mechanism of change. Acknowledging this problem, Hollon and Ponniah (2010) reviewed the randomized controlled psychotherapy trials for mood disorders. The authors identified 125 studies that included, among other treatments, emotion-focused therapy (the dynamically oriented treatment discussed in Chapter 1, developed by Greenberg, 2011), mindfulness-based therapies, brief psychodynamic therapies, and CBT (among others). For major depression, the results showed that CBT was efficacious and specific in the prevention of relapse/recurrence following treatment termination. Mindfulness-based therapy also appeared to be efficacious. However, the efficacy of emotion-focused therapy and brief psychodynamic therapies were less clear. Despite the specific names given to some of these treatments, it remains unclear for many of these interventions what exactly the treatment strategies are designed to do and whether they are, in fact, achieving the desired goal.

In order to examine the effect of specific strategies, such as reappraisal, on emotional response, it is necessary to examine the effects of this strategy in tightly controlled laboratory studies. A case in point is the cognitive model of social anxiety disorder. One of the concrete predictions of the model is that, when confronted with social threat, socially anxious individuals focus their attention inwardly onto negative self-focused cognitions, leading to heightened social anxiety and subsequent avoidance behaviors, resulting in the maintenance of the problem (Hofmann, 2007). Consistent with this model are correlational and mediation studies showing that successful treatment is mediated via changes in appraisal of social situations (Hofmann, 2004) and also associated with decreased self-focused attention (Hofmann, 2000; Wells & Papageorgiou, 1998) and improvements in self-perception (Hofmann, Moscovitch, Kim, & Taylor, 2004). Many laboratory studies also support the value of reappraisal techniques to alter emotional states. For example, in one study we assessed anxious responding in participants who anticipated public speaking (Schulz, Alpers, & Hofmann, 2008). To examine the role of cognitions as a mediator, we induced negative self-focused cognitions as compared with relaxation that encouraged participants to focus their attention away from negative cognitions. As predicted by the cognitive model, negative self-focused cognitions fully mediated the effects of trait social anxiety on self-reported anxiety and heart rate variability during negative anticipation. These and many other studies (e.g., Hofmann et al., 2013) support the basic idea that reappraisal directly influences emotional responding.

Summary of Clinically Relevant Points

- Emotions are not directly caused by an event or situation but by the maladaptive perception and interpretation (cognitive appraisal) of this event or situation.

- Overarching general beliefs, or schemas, about oneself, the world, and the future are at the core of the cognitive distortions about events or situations that give rise to maladaptive automatic cognitions.

- Emotional reasoning is a cognitive process that uses one's emotional experience (e.g., "I am anxious") as evidence for the validity of thought ("The situation must have been dangerous because I felt anxious"). This establishes a positive feedback loop that supports the belief by the experience.

- Cognitive biases are not necessarily unhealthy. Cognitions are unhealthy when they are maladaptive because they provide little assistance in adapting to life's challenges.

- Maladaptive schemas are relatively resistant to change because they often develop early in life and become characterological problems.

CHAPTER SEVEN

◆

Positive Affect and Happiness

The primary goal in clinical psychology, psychiatry, and related fields has been to reduce or eliminate the suffering in patients with negative affective states, such as depression and anxiety. Therefore, mental health research and practice has also been primarily focused on studying and reducing negative affect. In contrast, relatively little is known about strategies to enhance positive affect, despite the substantial body of literature underscoring the role that positive affect plays in the onset, overlap, and maintenance of anxiety and depression. Although positive and negative affect are negatively associated, the absence of negative affect does not necessarily, or even usually, lead to enhanced positive affect. This chapter discusses the role of positive affect and happiness in emotional disorders and describes strategies to enhance it.

DEFINING POSITIVE AFFECT AND HAPPINESS

Psychology researchers distinguish between two types of positive well-being: *hedonic* and *eudaimonic*. Hedonic well-being describes transient and positive feelings, such as happiness and contentment (e.g., Kahneman, Diener, & Schwarz, 2003), whereas eudaimonic well-being describes the enduring emotions that accompany movement toward one's own potential, such as feelings of vitality, curiosity, and engagement (e.g., Diener, 2000).

Positive affect and the feeling of happiness are elusive goals. People quickly adapt to new possessions, wealth, luxuries, and fame. A person who wins a few million dollars in a lottery will only report a high degree of happiness soon after winning. Over time, she will attribute considerably less happiness to her financial windfall. This has been termed the *law of hedonic asymmetry* by Frijda (1988) and is consistent with the notion of the *hedonic treadmill* (Brickman & Campbell, 1971). The hedonic treadmill turns happiness into an elusive state because expectations rise with one's possessions and accomplishments. Fortunately, unhappiness is similarly transient, because people also adapt to undesirable situations. We overestimate both the positive affect we expect to experience in response to a desirable future event and the negative affect we expect to experience in response to an undesirable future event. In other words, people's prospection, or *affective forecasting*, abilities tend to be biased because they tend to exaggerate their emotional response to an anticipated future event (Gilbert & Wilson, 2007).

The reason for this bias is, in part, that predictions are decontextualized. In other words, hedonic experiences are influenced by mental representations, as well as by contextual factors. The bias arises because people tend to overlook the fact that the contextual factors present when we make the predictions are not the same as the contextual factors that will be present when the event is actually happening. This is not just true for the prediction of happiness. For example, people who have just completed a strenuous exercise at a gym mistakenly predict that they would enjoy drinking water the next day more than do people who are about to begin their exercise (Van Boven & Loewenstein, 2003).

HISTORICAL BACKGROUND

Although studies of positive subjective experiences have appeared in the psychological literature only fairly recently and primarily under the rubric *positive psychology* (Seligman & Csikszentmihalyi, 2000), some of the relevant constructs have a long history and tradition. In particular, the construct of happiness has been the subject of many philosophies and religions throughout human history. Happiness is a central theme of Buddhist teachings. Ultimate happiness may be defined as *Nirvana* (or *Bodhi*), the state of everlasting peace, that is free from suffering, anger, and cravings (e.g., Buddhaghosa, 1975). The way for practitioners to reach this state of everlasting peace and cessation of suffering is through the *Noble Eightfold Path.* Similarly, the Chinese Confucian disciple Mencius, who lived in the third century B.C.E., believed that all people were born with the innate capacity to be good and happy. In contrast, Aristotle (who lived at around the same time as Mencius) believed humans must learn to acquire happiness through experience and practice. In his *Nicomachean Ethics,* he further proposed that happiness is the purpose of human nature and, therefore, the only state that humans desire for its own sake (rather than friendship, wealth, etc.).

More than a millennium later, Saint Thomas Aquinas (1225–1274) laid the foundation of the modern view of happiness by directly linking happiness to willful actions. Specifically, he assumed that, in order to reach happiness, an individual's will must be ordered toward the right goals and virtues. Aquinas agreed with Aristotle that happiness cannot be reached solely through reasoning about consequences of acts but that it also requires a pursuit of good causes for acts that are governed by natural or divine laws.

Similarly, later Western philosophers, and especially British ethicists, have argued that happiness is closely related to one's actions and their consequences. One philosophical principle directly speaks to this. This principle is known as *utilitarianism,* which states that we should always act in such a way that brings the most happiness and least unhappiness to oneself and other people.

Some of the main proponents of this principle were John Stuart Mill and Jeremy Bentham (Mill was Bentham's student). Bentham (1789/1988) understood happiness as a predominance of pleasure over pain. Thus, as an ethical hedonist, he believed that it is the amount of pleasure a specific action is likely going to cause that determines the rightness and wrongness of this action. He formulated an algorithm, the *felicific calculus,* to estimate the degree of pleasure a specific action is likely to cause. The variables that are considered in this algorithm include intensity and duration of the pleasure consequence, as well as how certain it is that the pleasurable consequence will happen, how quickly it will occur, how likely it is that the pleasurable consequence will be repeated in the future, and how many people will be affected by it. Bentham treated all forms of happiness as being basically equal. In contrast, Mill (1861/2001) argued that intellectual and moral pleasures are superior to the lower, more physical, forms of pleasures.

This brief excursion into the history of happiness illustrates the long tradition and complexity of the definition of the term and other forms of positive affect. The issues that are central to these emotional states are closely tied to some of the fundamental philosophical questions about human nature (e.g., What is the purpose of our existence?). I am not able to answer these questions here. Instead, I explore the function of happiness for mental health in general and for emotions in particular.

POSITIVE AFFECT IS NOT
THE ABSENCE OF NEGATIVE AFFECT

Positive and negative affect are not two poles on the same continuum. However, they are also not completely unrelated. Although negative affect features prominently in emotional disorders, positive affect is also an important, but less investigated, dimension. Research examining the hierarchical structure of emotional disorders reveals two primary dimensions: *neuroticism/negative affectivity* and *extraversion/positive affectivity* (Brown, 2007; Brown & Barlow, 2009; Clark & Watson, 1991). For example, a study by Brown and Barlow (2009) found that virtually all of the considerable covariance among latent variables corresponding to DSM-IV constructs of unipolar depression, generalized anxiety disorder, social anxiety disorder, obsessive–compulsive disorder, panic disorder, and agoraphobia was explained by the higher-order dimensions of negative and positive affect. Thus some emotional disorders are associated not only with heightened negative affect but also with lowered positive affect (Carl, Soskin, Kerns, & Barlow, 2013; Hofmann, Sawyer, Fang, & Asnaani, 2012).

Similar to negative affect, positive affect is not a constant experience. Both fluctuate over time and are influenced by a number of factors. Although positive and negative affect are not simply opposite ends of the same continuum, they are not completely independent, either; as one of them becomes stronger, the other becomes weaker.

The *broaden-and-build model* states that positive affect loosens the influence of negative affect on the person and at the same time broadens his or her behavioral repertoire by enhancing physical, social, and intellectual resources (e.g., Fredrickson, 2000). In other words, this model assumes positive affect is adaptive because it provides people with an opportunity to expand on their resources and social relationships to prepare for future challenges. As a result of the frequent experience of positive affect, happy people are generally also more successful (Lyubomirsky, King, & Diener, 2005) and have healthier lives. For example, a review of 26 prospective observational studies found that positive well-being was associated with reduced mortality (Chida & Steptoe, 2008). These effects persisted even when negative affect was taken into consideration. Therefore, negative and positive affect can coexist. Common examples are moments of joy and sadness, such as the happy father who cries during the wedding of his daughter. This study illustrates the importance of positive affect for health. Similarly, a 15-year prospective study with more than 11,000 individuals who were initially free of coronary heart disease found that those with greater psychological well-being had a markedly reduced risk of developing a coronary heart disease after accounting for other known risk factors (Kubzansky & Thurston, 2007).

MEASURING POSITIVE AFFECT AND HAPPINESS

Positive affect and happiness are difficult to measure reliably. Life satisfaction is a reasonable proxy measure for it. For example, it has been found that, among people who report that they are above neutral in their life satisfaction, the vast majority (85%) report that they feel happy at least half of the time (Lucas, Diener, & Suh, 1996). A frequently used direct measure of happiness is the Subjective Happiness Scale by Lyubomirsky and Lepper (1999). This scale includes four items that directly ask participants about their level of happiness on a 7-point scale. For example, item 1 asks each participant whether he or she considers him- or herself to be a generally happy person, and item 2 asks whether the person considers him- or herself to be more or less happy compared with most of his or her peers.

Happiness has been defined as a frequent experience of positive affect (Lyubomirsky et al., 2005). Therefore, some investigators assess positive affect as a proxy measure of happiness. A commonly used measure of positive affect is the Positive and Negative Affect Scale (PANAS; Watson, Clark, & Tellegen, 1988), which asks participants to indicate on a 1- (*very slightly* to *not at all*) to 5- (*extremely*) point scale how they feel at the present moment (or felt over the past week) using 10 positive (e.g., *interested, proud, active*) and 10 negative (e.g., *distressed, upset, scared*) adjectives. The scale provides a positive and a negative affect score (see also Appendix I). The positive affect score may, therefore, be considered as a measure of happiness. However, two people may essentially receive the same positive affect score but markedly different negative affect scores. Therefore, it could be argued that happiness is not only defined by high positive affect but also by low negative affect. This issue has been discussed as early as 1969 by Bradburn, who proposed an affect balance measure that is derived by subtracting negative affect from positive affect.

PREDICTING POSITIVE AFFECT AND HAPPINESS

It is difficult to identify reliable predictors or correlates of happiness and positive affect. Age, gender, and even money (beyond a minimum amount required to provide for basic needs of food and shelter) tend to be unreliable predictors (Myers & Diener, 1995). Rather than material wealth and luxury, very happy people have relatively rich and satisfying social relationships and spend little time alone. In contrast, unhappy people have poor social relationships. The happiest people show the lowest level of psychopathology, which is consistent with earlier views suggesting that depression is associated with low positive affect (Watson, Clark, & Mineka, 1994).

Although happy people in Diener and Seligman's (2002) sample reported feeling unpleasant emotions at certain times, they rarely felt euphoria or ecstasy. Instead, they felt medium to moderately strong pleasant emotions much of the time. These findings suggest that very happy people have the ability to move upward in mood without experiencing euphoria when good situations present themselves and that they are able to react with negative moods when something bad occurs (Diener & Seligman, 2002). Moreover, this study's results suggest that happiness is not associated with the intensity of positive affect but rather with the amount of time that people experience positive affect.

Happiness and life satisfaction are associated with a number of temperamental traits, including optimism, hardiness, and other characteristics of a person that promote positive feelings, such as hope and humor when confronted with difficult situations (e.g., Lyubomirsky et al., 2005). For example, a longitudinal study of Finnish twins showed that life satisfaction was associated with a lower risk of suicide 20 years later, even after controlling for a number of known risk factors, such as age, sex, smoking, physical activity, and substance use (Koivumaa-Honkanen et al., 2001)

WANDERING MINDS, UNHAPPY MINDS

Some people excessively ruminate about the past or worry about the future. Rumination is a characteristic feature of depression; worrying is a characteristic feature of many anxiety disorders, such as generalized anxiety disorder. But ruminating about the past and worrying about the future are not at all unique to these particular mental disorders; they are part of being human. Unlike other species, humans spend a lot of time thinking about past and possible future events. Insurance companies constitute a multi-billion-dollar industry that aims to give customers peace of mind; we spend large sums of money for our retirement and for our children's college education. Thus our minds are focused not only on the present moment but also on the past. This is to some extent also true for nonhuman species (e.g., animals prepare for the winter or build nests for their offspring). However, the degree of past- and future-oriented behaviors is considerably greater in humans than in other species. Moreover, it could be argued that nonhuman animals do not show the same degree of cognition as humans in anticipating future events but rather respond to stimuli in the environment that precede the future events (e.g., birds do not build their nests because they anticipate brooding but because seasonal changes and other factors activate an instinctual drive).

The ability of humans to anticipate future events (and to ruminate about the past) comes at an emotional cost, because thinking about places and times other than the present moment tend to make us feel unhappy; or as Killingsworth and Gilbert (2010) recently summarized it: *A wandering mind is an unhappy mind*. The authors conducted a study using an iPhone. An application on the iPhone contacted users at random moments during the day and asked them questions about what they are doing, how they were feeling, and whether their minds were wandering. More specifically, the study analyzed samples from 2,250 adults who answered questions on their current mood states (*How are you feeling right now?*), current activities (*What are you doing right now?*), and whether or not their minds were currently wandering (*Are you thinking about something other than what you're currently doing?*). The results showed that people's minds wandered often, regardless of what they were actually doing at the moment. Mind wandering happened in at least 30% of the data points taken during every activity, except for making love. People were less happy when their minds were wandering than when they were not. Interestingly, this was the case during all activities. Even when their minds wandered more to pleasant topics (42.5% of the samples) than to unpleasant topics (26.5%), people did not report being happier when thinking about something other than their current activities. The authors were also able to show that mind wandering was generally the cause rather than the consequence of unhappiness. Finally, it was shown that happiness was predicted by what people were thinking rather than by what people were doing. The authors concluded that "a human mind is a wandering mind, and a wandering mind is an unhappy mind. The ability to think about what is not happening is a cognitive achievement that comes at an emotional cost" (Killingsworth & Gilbert, 2010, p. 932). The reverse might also be true: being in the here and now, experiencing life in the present moment, mindfully, rather than dwelling about other things, such as ruminating about missed chances in the past or potential threat in the future, seems to be associated with psychological health and happiness.

MINDFULNESS

Mindfulness is a popular term that is discussed in a wide variety of fields, ranging from social (Langer, 1989) to clinical (Kabat-Zinn, 2003; Williams & Penman, 2011) areas. Many of the contemporary mindfulness exercises focus on breathing and present-moment awareness. As an example, Zen (Zazen) meditation, a traditional Japanese mediation practice that is rooted in Buddhism, consists solely of sitting meditation. Other techniques are intended to enhance different sensory experiences, such as sound, smell, taste, texture, or temperature. All of these strategies encourage the person to focus attention on a specific sensory experience. In addition to sensory meditation strategies, other exercises focus on the affective experience, as is the case with loving-kindness and compassion-focused meditation. These practices are described at a later point.

Historical Background

Historically, the term *mindfulness* is deeply rooted in Eastern philosophy, especially Buddhism, Zen, and Yoga. Buddhism dates back to Shakyamuni Buddha, who lived in India more than 2,500 years ago. His teachings spread across India, Sri Lanka, and Central Asia and reached China at around the first century C.E. There, early Buddhism merged with Taoism, Confucianism, and other religious cultures. Zen evolved through the merging of early Buddhism with Taoism and became the more modern form of Buddhist practices.

All Buddhist practices emphasize mindfulness. Key in the understanding of mindfulness is the role of suffering (*dukkha*) and the *Four Noble Truths* about suffering: (1) the truth of *dukkha* (i.e., the realization that suffering is a fact of life and unavoidable); (2) the truth of the origin of *dukkha*; (3) the truth of the cessation of *dukkha*; and (4) the truth of overcoming *dukkha*. The suffering can be due to physical and mental illness, growing old, and the stress of trying to hold onto things that are constantly changing.

Buddhism, also referred to as Buddha-dharma, emphasizes that through the practice of *dharma* it is possible to overcome suffering and attain peace and happiness, as well as purification and enlightenment, a state of being in which hatred, greed, and other negative feelings are overcome. *Dharma* refers here to a way of living a life of high morals and values consistent with the teachings of Buddha. In Buddhism, these lifestyles and practices are often referred to as the *path of purification*, leading to the *path of enlightenment*. Similar ideas can be found in Yoga and other Eastern traditions, such as Zen. Thus, for many, mindfulness is not limited to meditation practices but also includes a lifestyle characterized by calmness and awareness of one's own body and of one's feelings and thoughts. Mindfulness brings the person into harmony with reality and avoids ignorance and self-inflicted suffering, which are considered to be the chief obstacle to happiness. In Buddhism, ignorance means viewing oneself as separate from others and the world. In contrast, Buddhism emphasizes the connectedness between oneself and everything else.

The opposite of mindfulness is the failure to see and accept reality and the true nature of things as they are. Thus the Buddhist view of our situation in life is neither pessimistic nor optimistic but realistic—which, incidentally, is consistent with the generic CBT model. Failure to see the true nature of things is expressed as ignorance (*avijja*) and delusion (*moha*). Ignorance is sometimes distinguished between two interrelated types: ignorance of the true nature of things and the ignorance of the laws of karma and interdependence, which then results in an inaccurate relationship to the world. Both types of ignorance lead to the inability to recognize one's fullest capacity and can result in doubt, stubbornness, and emotional distress. The antidote to ignorance is wisdom—the ability to know and correctly perceive.

Defining Mindfulness

Mindfulness is difficult to define and measure, but relatively easy to practice. Numerous studies have found that mindfulness practices are effective for treating a variety of emotional disorders, especially mood and anxiety problems. The precise mechanism is not completely understood.

Mindfulness, generally speaking, refers to both a state of attentive present-moment awareness of reality and a set of procedures for achieving that state. The contemporary literature defines *mindfulness* as a process that leads to a mental state characterized by nonjudgmental awareness of the present-moment experience, including one's thoughts, bodily sensations, consciousness, and the environment, while encouraging openness, curiosity, and acceptance (Bishop et al., 2004; Kabat-Zinn, 2003; Langer & Moldoveanu, 2000; Melbourne Academic Mindfulness Interest Group, 2006). Mindfulness strategies focus on the present moment, encouraging people to pay attention to it without judging it.

Bishop and colleagues (2004) distinguish two components of mindfulness, one that involves self-regulation of attention and one that involves an orientation toward the present moment characterized by openness, curiosity, and acceptance. The basic premise underlying mindfulness practices is that experiencing the present moment nonjudgmentally and openly can effectively counter the effects of stressors, because excessive orientation toward the past or future when dealing with stressors can lead to (or reinforce) depression and anxiety symptoms (e.g., Kabat-Zinn, 2003). It is further believed that, by teaching people to respond to stressful situations more reflectively rather than reflexively, mindfulness practice can effectively counter experiential avoidance strategies, which are attempts to alter the intensity or frequency of unwanted internal experiences (Hayes et al., 2006). These avoidance strategies are believed to contribute to the maintenance of many, if not all, emotional disorders (Bishop et al., 2004; Hayes, 2004). In addition, the slow breathing involved in mindfulness meditation may alleviate bodily symptoms of distress by balancing sympathetic and parasympathetic responses (Kabat-Zinn, 2003).

Mindfulness training might be conceived of as a multistage attention training process. In the initial stages, mindfulness practice heightens one's awareness of reactive processes; in the middle stages, it leads to the disengagement of automatic reactivity specific to the targeted experience; in the final stage, it supports the emergence of more integrative response potentials and self-acceptance in domains of functioning (Kristeller, 2007). Similarly, Hölzel and colleagues (2011) propose that attention regulation is an important aspect. In addition, they consider body awareness, emotion regulation, and change in perspective on the self as important components that determine the mechanism of change. Finally, DeSteno and his team reported evidence to suggest that mindfulness training increases compassionate and prosocial behaviors (Condon, Desbordes, Miller,

& DeSteno, 2013; Lim, Condon, & DeSteno, 2015). However, despite these promising findings, the precise mechanisms of mindfulness and their neurobiological correlates are poorly understood.

Nevertheless, mindfulness practices are clinically useful because they seem to effectively target maladaptive cognitive processes, such as worrying and ruminating, in effect to generate distance between one's thoughts and one's perception of self (often resulting in the real-ization "I am not my thoughts"). Being mindful means being in the present moment rather than thinking about the past or future events or thinking about issues that are unrelated to the present moment. Being mindful also means experiencing the emotions associated with the current state. Although many mindfulness practices focus on pleasant experiences, the goal of mindfulness exercises is not to feel good. Rather, mindfulness practices encourage the person to be open minded and curious, to experience whatever is indeed going on, without judging it or trying to change it. In contrast, mindless actions are automatic and affect-free, or even associated with negative affect. Interestingly, as I discuss later, there is a direct relationship between the degree of mindfulness and affect.

Distancing and Decentering

Mindfulness in sensory meditation practices (i.e., practices focused on breathing and other sensory experiences) exercises the patient's voluntary attentional processes. These sensory meditation strategies encourage the person to focus on the present moment rather than on past or future events and to develop a nonjudgmental stance toward any experiences, thoughts, and feelings. This process is also often referred to as *decentering*, which is closely related to the concept of *distancing* in traditional CBT (Beck, 1970). Although these two concepts are highly overlapping, both conceptually and practically, there are also some subtle differences between them, especially in their respective theoretical foundations. Distancing refers to the pro-cess of gaining objectivity toward thoughts by learning to distinguish between thoughts and reality. Distancing assumes knowledge can be achieved by evaluating one's thoughts, which may be expressed in the form of hypotheses. In contrast, decentering, as it is used by some authors (e.g., Hayes, 2004), assumes a theoretical model that does not make a distinction between thoughts and behaviors on a conceptual level, because thoughts are conceived as verbal behaviors.

The inability of a person to engage in decentering and distancing can result in *thought–action fusion* (TAF), which refers to the difficulty of separating cognitions from behaviors. It has been proposed that TAF comprises two discrete components (Shafran, Thordarson, & Rachman, 1996). The first component is the belief that experiencing a particular thought increases the chance that an event will actually occur (likelihood), whereas the second component (morality) is the belief that thinking about an action is tantamount to performing the action. For example, for someone involved in TAF, the thought of killing another person may be considered morally equivalent to actually killing that person. Shafran and colleagues (1996) assume that the moral component is the result of the erroneous conclusion that experiencing "bad" thoughts is indicative of one's "true" nature and intentions.

Mindfulness is an activity that can be taught and practiced. It is also a trait and interindividual difference variable associated with adaptive emotional responding, as shown in some recent experimental studies. For example, in a study by Arch and Craske (2010), participants were assessed in response to a hyperventilation stressor. Trait mindfulness was associated with diminished responses to this stressor in samples with and without clinical anxiety. Another study found that trait mindfulness predicted less reactivity to a hyperventilation task in individuals both with and without anxiety. In this study, trait mindfulness was found to predict lower cortisol responses and less subjective distress to a social evaluative threat (Brown, Weinstein, & Creswell, 2012). Finally, it has been found that trait mindfulness can buffer the maladaptive effects of suppressing unpleasant emotions (Bullis et al., 2014). In this study, we trained participants to use a suppression strategy and then instructed them to suppress their responses to the inhalation of a 15% CO_2-enriched air mixture. After controlling for anxiety-related variables, trait mindfulness was the only significant predictor of the distress associated with the unpleasant emotions that arose from suppressing the bodily sensations caused by the inhalation of CO_2-enriched air. More specifically, the ability to provide descriptions of observed experiences predicted less heart rate reactivity to CO_2 inhalation, whereas skillfulness at restricting attention to the present moment was uniquely predictive of less subjective distress. The tendency to attend to bodily or sensory stimuli predicted greater distress during CO_2 inhalation. These recent laboratory studies point to the importance of trait mindfulness as a buffer for dealing with stressful situations.

Mindfulness-Based Therapies

Mindfulness-based therapies have gained enormous popularity and shown potential benefits. Popular examples of mindfulness-based therapy (MBT) include mindfulness-based cognitive therapy (MBCT; e.g., Segal et al, 2002) and mindfulness-based stress reduction (MBSR; e.g., Kabat-Zinn, 1982). Meta-analytic reviews have shown that mindfulness-based interventions are effective for treating depression and anxiety (Hofmann, Sawyer, Witt, & Oh, 2010; Khoury et al., 2013). Other studies have shown that MBT is also effective for a variety of psychological problems and is especially effective for reducing anxiety, depression, and stress (e.g., Carmody & Baer, 2009; Grossman, Niemann, Schmidt, & Walach, 2004).

MINDFUL SITTING AND BREATHING

Mindfulness exercises include training attention to interrupt automaticity, slow down one's thoughts, and intensify one's experience of being in the here and now. A commonly used exercise is mindful sitting and breathing.

In Practice: Mindful Sitting and Breathing

For the typical sitting meditation practice, the patient is encouraged to find a private, clean, orderly, and quiet place without any distractions. It should not be too cold or too warm and not too dark or too bright. The basic instructions are as follows:

1. *Wear loose and comfortable clothes. You should not be hungry, not too full, and not intoxicated. Sit on a pillow with your knees on the floor. It also helps to have a thick mat underneath. Cross your legs in either the half or full lotus position and sit up straight. Put your hands on your upper legs and fold one*

hand into the palm of the other. Keep your eyes slightly open, without focusing on any particular object. Keep your mouth closed and place your tongue against the roof of your month.

2. Breathe quietly through your nose in the way it feels most comfortable to you (do not try to control it by breathing very deeply or shallowly). Simply let breathing happen to you.

3. Do not try to control your thoughts or focus on any particular object. Let your thoughts come and go. Be aware of your own and others' presence, the surroundings, and any sensations, including your breathing and your posture.

4. The goal is to heighten awareness, not to reach a state of drowsiness. Typically the practices are done daily at around the same time of day, and each practice is usually 20–40 minutes long. Start with 10 minutes or so and slowly increase the time.

MINDFUL EATING

Eating is driven by a basic motivation. Our bodies are equipped with a number of feedback mechanisms that determine when we should start eating, when we should stop eating, and what we should eat. These feedback cues can be subtle, and disruptions in these mechanisms can lead to disordered eating behaviors.

In addition to serving our physical needs, eating also has an important social function in virtually all human cultures; humans gather to eat to celebrate important milestones, ranging from weddings and birthdays to graduations and funerals. Even prisoners on death row are offered a last meal before being executed, underscoring the powerful role of eating as a biological, social, and emotional reinforcer.

Despite the importance humans place on eating together on certain occasions, meals can be of secondary importance during our daily lives. Eating meals can become a nuisance and a necessary method of relieving unpleasant feelings of hunger. Fast-food restaurants are popular because they satisfy the basic hunger instinct in the fastest and least expensive way possible.

In addition, eating can be used as a way to regulate emotions, ranging from eating "comfort food" to the aberrant eating in bulimia nervosa, anorexia nervosa, and obesity. Eating can be used as a way to exert control over others or to express political opinions, such as in the case of hunger strikes. Finally, eating can develop into a habit or a way of enhancing other behaviors, such as munching popcorn while watching a movie.

Eating fulfills many different functions aside from simply satisfying one's hunger. It can be motivated by instinct (to satisfy hunger), or it may be used as way to regulate emotions (as in the case of bulimia nervosa, bulimia, and some forms of obesity). Eating can be mindless, habitual, and automatic (as in the case of munching popcorn in a movie), or it can be mindful and sensation-oriented (i.e., eating itself, with all its pleasant and possibly unpleasant experiences, is at the center of one's attention). Mindless eating is often habitual and fast, and it often serves an emotion-regulation function. In contrast, mindful eating is deliberate, slow, and sensation-focused to enhance awareness of hunger, the texture and taste of food, the act of chewing and swallowing, and feelings of satiation. Mindful eating can also include considerations and contemplations about the nature, origin, and processing of the food. For example, when eating an apple, one might imagine the farmer who harvested it or the tree that carried it and the blossom that attracted the bee that pollinated it.

These considerations are consistent with Buddhist views of interrelations of all living beings and can enhance the appreciation of the eating experience. These practices are obviously easier when there is no time pressure and when the food is tasty and fresh rather than highly processed and bland or greasy.

When practicing mindful eating, it is advised to initially avoid sour- or bitter- tasting foods, such as lemon or grapefruit, and highly processed food, such as caramel candy bars, and hard food items, such as nuts and celery. The ideal food item, especially at the beginning, is something that is familiar and that does not require a lot of chewing. Ideally, it should create a longer-lasting pleasant gustatory experience, such as a banana or a raisin. Later exercises may include food that is associated with a more complex texture, such as dark chocolate, apples, grapes, cheese, or bread. The following instructions can enhance the mindful eating experience.

In Practice: Mindful Eating

Mindful eating can enhance the experience of savoring food. By focusing on the subtleties of the eating experience, we resist the urge to race through a meal. This enhances the satisfaction eating is typically associated with, but also makes us more aware of the subtle cues that signal us to stop eating or to pause. Instructions might include the following:

Explore the food. Look at the food item as if you're seeing it for the first time; move it across your lips to experience its texture and temperature, smell it. Slowly put it in your mouth and concentrate on the sensations it creates. With your tongue, slowly experience the texture and taste. Notice your saliva surrounding it and notice how the experience changes as you slowly chew it. Notice your impulse to swallow it. Slowly swallow it and notice the change in taste and texture as you continue eating the food item.

As you are eating it, think about the origin of the food item and how many living beings were involved in this experience. For example, if you are eating an apple, think about the apple tree that carried the fruit. Think about the bees that pollinated the blossom; think about the farmer who picked the apples and the grocery store workers who handled the apple.

Additional instructions to further enhance the experience may include the following:

1. *Avoid taking big bites; experiment with eating with chopsticks because you will have less food per bite.*

2. *Experiment with eating with your nondominant hand; it enhances the eating experience, and less food per bite enters your mouth.*

3. *Chew a lot; for example, you may try to chew 30–50 times per bite; make the meal last at least 20 minutes.*

4. *Avoid any distractions, such as TV, newspapers, or computers.*

5. *Put less food on your plate than you feel you want to eat.*

Mindfulness activities are not restricted to sitting, breathing, and eating. Any activity can be turned from an automatic mindless task into a mindful experience (e.g., Langer, 1989). Driving to work, drinking wine, having sex, and so forth can be done in a mindless or in a mindful way while focusing on the different sensations and experiences, especially the pleasurable aspects. If an activity is done in a mindful way, it generates more intense and typically also more positive affect than if it is done in a mindless and automatic way. Mindfulness takes time and practice. Regular mindfulness training can turn routine, normal, and automatic activities into meaningful, mindful ones.

LOVING-KINDNESS AND COMPASSION MEDITATION

Mindfulness meditation exercises that are known to most Westerners encourage nonjudgmental awareness of experiences in the present moment. Compassion meditation (CM) also requires mindfulness, but the focus of attention is not directed only toward sensory experiences but on the awareness and wish to alleviate the suffering of all living and conscious (i.e., sentient) beings. In loving-kindness meditation (LKM), the focus is on loving and kind concern for the well-being of others. LKM aims to develop an affective state of unconditional kindness to all people. LKM is particularly useful for enhancing positive affect. Because *loving kindness* is an unusual term that can elicit some resistance, an alternative description might be the term *positive affect training.*

LKM and CM (as well as sympathetic joy and equanimity) are seen as attributes that underlie the nonjudgmental aspect of mindful awareness because, without them, negative judgments can interfere with sustained mindfulness. For this reason, LKM and CM both include the practice of mindfulness. The aim of LKM is to develop an affective state of unconditional kindness to all people. CM aims to cultivate a deep, genuine sympathy for people who have encountered misfortune, together with an earnest wish to ease this suffering (for a review, see Feldman, 2005; Hofmann, Grossman, & Hinton, 2011; Hopkins, 2001; Salzberg, 1995).

These meditation practices are believed to broaden attention, enhance positive affect, and lessen negative affective states. They are believed to shift a person's basic view of the self in relation to others and increase empathy and compassion (Dalai Lama & Cutler, 1998). In traditional Buddhist practices, LKM is considered particularly helpful for people who have a strong tendency toward hostility or anger (e.g., Anālayo, 2003; Sheng-Yen, 2001).

Historical Background

Loving-kindness, also known as *metta* (in Pali), is derived from Buddhism. It refers to a mental state of unselfish and unconditional kindness to all beings (Dalai Lama, 2001). Compassion (*karunaa*) can be defined as an emotion that elicits the wish that people be free from suffering and the causes of suffering (Hopkins, 2001).

In the Buddhist tradition, LKM and CM have been combined with other meditation practices, especially mindfulness meditation. Loving-kindness and compassion are closely linked to the Buddhist notion that all living beings are inextricably connected. Together with loving-kindness and compassion, sympathetic joy (*mutida*; i.e., joy in the other's joy, the opposite of schadenfreude) and equanimity (*upekkha*; being calm and even-tempered) constitute the four *brahma-viharas*. These are regarded as four sublime states (also known as noble and divine abodes or "immeasurables"); for more details, see Buddhaghosa (1975). These four attitudinal qualities form the foundation of the Buddhist ethical system and are seen as characteristics necessary to achieve insight into the workings of our own minds and the world around us and to attain a life free from misery. According to the Buddhist view, in order to effectively pay moment-to-moment attention to the perceptible (an inherently cognitive act), one needs to cultivate these four qualities. Without their presence when confronted by unpleasant or negative perceptions (e.g., negative self-thoughts, disturbing emotions, or distressing images), Buddhists believe the person would most likely enter an evaluative or ruminative state of mind. In that state of mind, the person would be unable to experience his or her emotional state as an object of attention and mindful awareness. Thus Buddhists believe that only when we are able to confront difficult sensations, emotions, or thoughts with a degree of kindness, compassion, and composure can we attend to the variety and textures of present-moment experiences in a mindful way.

Meditation Techniques

Buddhist practices often combine LKM and CM. Similarly, most psychological studies combined both approaches (Hofmann, Grossman, & Hinton, 2011; Lutz, Greischar, Perlman, & Davidson, 2009). In the elaborated form of compassion meditation, the person who meditates conducts a series of "contemplations" (i.e., thoughts). According to Buddhist tradition (Book 1, *uraga vagga* [the snake book], *cunda kammaraputta sutta* [AN 10.176]), at each stage the meditation exercise consists of thinking about specific aspirations (wishes) for another person, including the following: (1) may the person be free from enmity; (2) may the person be free from mental suffering; (3) may the person be free from physical suffering; and (4) may the person take care of him- or herself happily (see, e.g., Chalmers, 2007; Dalai Lama, 2001). Typically, the exercise begins by directing this feeling of compassion toward oneself or toward specific others, depending on what is easiest. Similarly, during LKM, the person typically proceeds from easier to more challenging types of contemplation. Typically, the feeling is extended to an ever-widening circle of others, ultimately radiating in all directions (north, south, east, and west), although the order can be changed to accommodate individual preferences.

When practicing LKM, the person gently repeats certain phrases in order to direct a positive energy of feeling, called *metta*, toward other people, as well as oneself. *Metta* refers to a mental state of unselfish and unconditional kindness to all beings. The phrases should not be used as a mantra that loses its meaning with repetition. Rather, the phrases are intended to keep one's attentional focus on *metta* and the target of it. Therefore, the phrases should be used mindfully each time, bringing one's full awareness to the phrases, their meaning, and the feelings they bring up. LKM is based on the Buddhist notion that all living beings are connected and happiness is derived from knowing our connection with all beings.

LKM can be practiced at any time and in different postures, such as when sitting, lying, or walking (Buddharakkhita, 1995; Dalai Lama, 2001). However, it is best to practice it while sitting comfortably in a quiet place with no distractions. The practices can be quite simple in their rudimentary forms. They typically include directing these feelings toward oneself, toward specific others, or in all directions to all beings.

In Practice: Loving-Kindness Meditation to Enhance Positive Affect

During LKM, the person typically proceeds from easier to more challenging types of contemplation (Buddharakkhita, 1995; Dalai Lama, 2001). A typical sequence is the following:

1. Focus on the self.
2. Focus on a "benefactor" or good friend (i.e., a person who is still alive and who does not invoke sexual desires).
3. Focus on a neutral person (i.e., a person who typically does not elicit either particularly positive or negative feelings but who is commonly encountered during a normal day).
4. Focus on a "difficult" person (i.e., a person who is typically associated with negative feelings).
5. Focus on the self, the good friend, the neutral person, and the difficult person (with attention being equally divided between them).
6. Focus on all beings east, west, north, and south and the entire universe.

These practices should not be seen as mere mechanical repetitions of images or phrases. Instead, by mindfully investigating what occurs when one attempts to generate loving-kindness or compassion, it is assumed that insight is gained into the nature of these emotions themselves, as well as one's personal relationships to them. Furthermore, by turning toward this focus of experience in a kind, open, patient, and tolerant manner, a shift in these affective states toward greater loving-kindness and compassion is thought to occur.

The most important goal is generating *metta*, an energy-like form of positive affect. The particular object that is targeted in this exercise is rather secondary. For example, alternatives to a "benefactor" may be a beloved pet or a friend from one's childhood, and a "neutral person" might be a cashier at a grocery store. When focusing on a difficult person, the patient should begin with a person with whom the difficulty is relatively mild; for example, someone mildly irritating or annoying rather than on a person who has hurt the patient deeply.

Note that practicing LKM toward a difficult person does not excuse this person's actions. Although forgiveness is a natural consequence of these practices, it is not the primary focus at the beginning. Similarly, it is not the goal to "like" the person; the goal is simply to wish the person happiness, embracing the realization that all people deserve to live a happy life without any suffering. In contrast, wishing people unhappiness leads to unhappiness in one's own life. In the words of the Dalai Lama, "Harboring anger towards another person is like swallowing poison and expecting another person to die." This is consistent with the Buddhist tradition that conceptualizes *metta* and *karuna* as being the two *brahma viharas* that are incompatible with anger, hatred, envy, and jealousy. Angry people are unhappy people, and true happiness is never self-centered but is always radiant and inclusive, because all beings are connected, and all humans are part of common humanity. This is emphasized when reflecting on the realization that all beings, including oneself, want to be happy (e.g., Salzberg, 1995).

Empirical Evidence

Both meditation practices have only recently been investigated in psychological experiments (Carson et al., 2005; Fredrickson et al., 2008; Hutcherson, Seppala, & Gross, 2008). Related to loving-kindness and compassion is the construct of *self-compassion*, which refers to compassion toward one's own suffering. It involves generating the desire to alleviate one's own suffering, healing oneself with kindness, recognizing one's shared humanity, and being mindful when considering negative aspects of oneself (Gilbert & Procter, 2006; Leary, Tate, Adams, Allen, & Hancock, 2007; Mayhew & Gilbert, 2008; Neff, 2003; Neff & Vonk, 2009).

The empirical evidence suggests that elements of LKM and CM can be trained within a relatively short period of time. For example, the study by Hutcherson and colleagues (2008) suggests that even a 7-minute training in LKM can produce small or moderately strong improvements in positive feelings toward strangers and oneself. However, the LKM training period will likely require more time. In other studies with nonclinical populations, the training consisted of six 60-minute weekly sessions (Fredrickson et al., 2008; Pace et al., 2009, 2010). The LKM exercise itself was only 15–20 minutes long (e.g., Fredrickson et al., 2008), although the effects were also modest. In clinical studies, the LKM training consisted of 12 weekly 2-hour sessions for treating anxiety, anger, and mood problems using a modification of CM (Gilbert & Procter, 2006), 12 weekly 1-hour sessions for treating paranoid symptoms in patients with schizophrenia (Mayhew & Gilbert, 2008), and 8 weekly 1-hour sessions to reduce chronic low back pain (Carson et al., 2005). Thus LKM and CM can have a positive effect on emotions and psychological functioning even after a relatively short period of training time.

It should be noted, however, that examining the effects of very short-term trainings focused on positive attention will not have the same effects as systematic trainings in which people spend many hours in LKM or CM directed toward themselves, loved ones, or even enemies. The basic Buddhist assumption is that these abilities take considerable time and practice to develop, and examining the effects of these practices in a laboratory by giving brief instructions to novices goes against that basic assumption. Therefore, it is quite possible that the trainings have very different effects when comparing novices with experts who have practiced for decades (as in the studies by Lutz, Slagter, Dunne, & Davidson, 2008; Lutz et al., 2009).

Finally, it is quite likely that CM and LKM techniques require integration with mindfulness practices to establish concentration and attention required for LKM and CM (Anālayo, 2003; Pandita, 1992; Sheng-Yen, 2001; Dalai Lama, 2001). When effects of LKM were examined alone in an intervention trial (Fredrickson et al., 2008), the effects on positive affect were significant but small. Future research is necessary to examine CM and especially LKM in a larger randomized controlled trial.

To conclude, the research literature so far suggests that LKM and CM are highly promising techniques for improving positive affect and also for reducing stress and negative affect such as anxiety and mood symptoms. LKM seems to be particularly useful for targeting interpersonal problems such as anger control issues. Moreover, CM and LKM appear to be particularly useful for treating relationship problems, such as marital conflicts, or counteracting the challenges among caregiving professions or nonprofessionals who must provide long-term care to a relative or friend.

Summary of Clinically Relevant Points

- Psychiatry has primarily been focusing on reducing negative affect, but very little effort has been made to raise positive affect. People differ in the degree to which they experience negative and positive affect. Positive affect is associated with happiness, vitality, and well-being.

- Happiness and positive affect are difficult to predict. However, these emotional states do, in turn, predict physical and mental health.

- Mindfulness is difficult to define. It refers to the mental process of distancing oneself from one's own thoughts. It is defined as the process that leads to a mental state characterized by nonjudgmental awareness of the present-moment experience, including one's sensations, thoughts, bodily states, consciousness, and the environment, while encouraging openness, curiosity, and acceptance.

- Being mindful means being in the present moment rather than thinking about the past or future events or thinking about issues that are unrelated to the present moment. In contrast, mindless actions are automatic and affect-free or even associated with negative affect, as is the case in mind wandering.

- Mindfulness trainings are exercises aimed at experiencing the present moment nonjudgmentally and openly. These exercises have been shown to be effective for dealing with ruminative and worrisome thinking styles that are typical in depression and anxiety.

- Loving-kindness and compassion meditation (LKM and CM, respectively) can promote both temporary and long-lasting feelings of happiness and positive affect. These meditative practices can also lessen negative affective states, shift a person's basic view of the self in relation to others, and increase empathy.

- CM and LKM may be particularly useful for treating anger control issues, depression, and dysthymia, as well as relationship problems, such as marital conflicts, or for counteracting the challenges among caregiving professions or nonprofessionals who must provide long-term care to a relative or friend.

CHAPTER EIGHT

◆

Neurobiology of Emotions

A review of the neurobiological correlates of emotions would easily fill a separate volume, with entire chapters covering different emotional states. Therefore, a brief review such as I can provide here is necessarily selective and incomplete. In this review, I primarily discuss the biological correlates of the topics that I covered in the previous chapters. More specifically, some of the questions I address are: What brain structures are linked to emotions and emotion regulation? What is the relationship between emotions and cognitions on the neurobiological level? And how do individuals differ on the neurobiological level? I concentrate primarily on the neurobiological correlates of fear and anxiety, because most neuropsychological investigations of emotions have focused on the neurocircuitry of fear and related emotional states.

NEUROBIOLOGICAL SYSTEMS OF EMOTIONS

Jeffrey Gray first formulated an influential neuropsychological theory of anxiety, which has undergone certain modifications and clarifications during subsequent years (Gray, 1987, 1990) and which was recently updated (Gray & McNaughton, 1996). Although primarily focused on anxiety, his theory had wide-reaching implications for emotion research because it emphasizes the importance of context and expectancies. In essence, Gray's model postulates the existence of three different fundamental neuropsychological systems in the mammalian brain: the behavioral approach system, the fight-or-flight system, and the behavioral inhibition system (BIS). The subjective experience of "fear" is, according to Gray's theory, most closely related to the fight-or-flight system, whereas "anxiety" is considered to be the result of the BIS. In the context of Gray's theory, the fight-or-flight system is activated by unconditioned punishment and nonreward, whereas the BIS is activated by signals of punishment or nonreward (i.e., by conditioned stimuli), innate stimuli, and novel stimuli. It has been hypothesized that high BIS sensitivity (Fowles, 1993) or an overactive BIS (Quay, 1988, 1993) would result in greater behavioral responsivity to impending punishment cues and, therefore, greater susceptibility to anxiety or depressive disorders. Although Gray's theory has been influential among anxiety researchers, it has relatively limited relevance to other emotional states in humans and for clinical practice.

More recent studies have focused on the amygdala as an important brain structure involved in processing of emotions, especially fear. These studies have shown that aversive stimulation consistently activates a subcortical pathway from the thalamus to amygdaloid nuclei (e.g., Davis & Whalen, 2001; LeDoux, 2000). It appears that there are separate branching circuits either through the central gray, mediating somatic emotional responses (expressed as the "freezing response" in the rat) or through the lateral region of the hypothalamus, leading to autonomic arousal. Once established, this neural network can influence other associated behavior because conditioned stimuli activate this same fear circuit.

LeDoux and others have shown from animal experiments that the amygdala is particularly important for processing and expressing emotions (e.g., LeDoux, 2000). LeDoux's model assumes that emotional cues are processed in two different ways, which differ in the speed and depth of processing. First, the visual information of a potentially threatening object projects to the visual thalamus, which is the central relay station of the visual sensory input, and then directly to the amygdala, which has close connections to the autonomic nervous system. The input can trigger the fight-or-flight response system with little or no conscious awareness. LeDoux (2000) named this process the *low road* to the amygdala because the process happens without higher cortical involvement. In addition to this subcortical process, it is assumed that the information is also sent from the thalamus to the visual cortex, which further processes the information. Higher cortical processes can inhibit the activation of the amygdala, suppressing the initial fight-or-flight response. Because this path to the amygdala involves higher cortical centers, LeDoux (2000) referred to it as the *high road* to the amygdala. This means that the fight-or-flight response is an automatic response that is primarily driven by subcortical brain structure. Higher cortical areas can suppress this process, but they cannot prevent it from happening. However, it is important to note that in humans it is possible to have emotions in the absence of an amygdala. For example, people with the Urbach–Wiethe syndrome, a rare recessive genetic disorder seen primarily in people living in the northern part of South Africa, show a successive degeneration of the amygdala, but they still show fear and other emotions. This suggests that fear and other emotions can be experienced even without the amygdala.

More recently, LeDoux (2015) presented a very different and significantly refined view of the neurobiological correlates of emotions. Most neuroscience research to date has made the implicit assumption that the basic neurocircuitry identified in the rodent brain when the animal is exposed to threat, for example, directly translates to human emotions, such as fear or anxiety. In his book, LeDoux convincingly argues that this approach is seriously flawed, because an emotion is by definition a conscious experience. Although the basic and unconscious processes observed in animal studies contribute to emotional feelings in humans, these processes should not be equated with emotional processes. This view is generally consistent with the approach toward emotions I have adopted in this book, as described in detail in Chapter 4 and elsewhere.

Human studies suggest that brain areas located at the front of the neocortex (i.e., the prefrontal areas), especially those in the ventral (front), dorsal (back), and lateral (side) areas are especially implicated in emotions. Particularly important neurobiological correlates of emotions seem to be the ventral portions of the prefrontal cortex (PFC) (which are typically implicated in language or response inhibition), the dorsal portions of the PFC (which are implicated in working memory and selective attention), the dorsal portions of the anterior cingulate cortex (ACC) (which are implicated in monitoring control processes), the dorsal portions of the medial PFC (which are implicated in reflecting upon one's own or someone else's affective states), and the insula (which receives viscerosensory inputs and appears to play a general role in affective experience; for a review, see Ochsner & Gross, 2008).

Neuroscientists have primarily examined these neurocircuits of emotions (particularly fear) by studying rats in the laboratory. A common paradigm in studying fear is to administer an electric shock together with other stimuli. The human analogue of this setup is the eye-blink startle paradigm (e.g., see Lang, Bradley, & Cuthbert, 1990). During the so-called *fear-potentiated startle paradigm*, people are presented with a loud noise through a headset while measuring the strength of the eye-blink startle response to this noise. The eye-blink to the noise can be measured with an electromyogram and is used as a measure of fear. The eye-blink response is stronger (potentiated) when people are in a fearful state (e.g., when exposed to unpleasant and fear-producing pictures). Other laboratory experiments that examine emotion regulation in humans involve presenting participants with emotional stimuli, such as pictures and movie clips, and giving them specific instructions to "handle their emotions" while monitoring their brain activity.

NEUROBIOLOGY OF EMOTION REGULATION

Human experiments have identified many brain areas that are involved in emotion regulation. For example, in one experiment, healthy women were presented with neutral pictures (e.g., a lamp) or negatively valenced pictures (e.g., a mutilated body) while they were lying in a functional magnetic resonance imaging (fMRI) scanner that measured their brain activation (Ochsner, Bunge, Gross, & Gabrieli, 2002). The women were instructed to view the picture and fully experience any emotional response it might elicit. The picture remained on the screen for an additional period of time with the instructions either to simply look at it or to reappraise the stimulus. As part of the reappraisal instructions, the women were asked to reinterpret the negative picture so that it no longer generated the negative affective response (e.g., the picture of the mutilated body is part of a horror movie that is not real). As predicted by LeDoux's (2000) model, reappraisal of the negative pictures reduced their negative affect (i.e., the women reported less negative affect) and was associated with increased activity in higher cortical structures (including the dorsal and ventral regions of the left lateral PFC and the dorsal medial PFC and decreased activity in the amygdala). Furthermore, increased activation in the ventrolateral PFC was correlated with decreased activation in the amygdala, suggesting that this part of the PFC may play an important role in conscious and voluntary regulation of emotional processes.

A number of reviews of human studies have described the relationships among subcortical regions involved in emotional reactivity, including the amygdala and cortical regions involved in emotion regulation (e.g., Davidson, Jackson, & Kalin, 2000; LeDoux, 2000; Ochsner & Gross, 2008). Abnormal fear responding can be a result of overactivity of the amygdala and abnormalities in prefrontal control, among other structures (e.g., Beck, 2008). Effective CBT can resolve these abnormalities (e.g., Clark & Beck, 2010; DeRubeis, Siegle, & Hollon, 2008).

Reappraisal is cognitively complex and requires processes necessary for generating, maintaining, and implementing a cognitive frame, as well as processes that track changes in one's emotional states. In a summary of the neuroimaging literature, Ochsner and Gross (2008) conclude that reappraisal is associated with activations of the ventral portions of the PFC (which are typically implicated in language or response inhibition), the dorsal portions of the PFC (which are implicated in working memory and selective attention), dorsal portions of the ACC (which are implicated in monitoring control processes), and dorsal portions of the medial PFC (which are implicated in reflecting upon one's own or someone else's affective states). Moreover, reappraisal seems to modulate systems involved in different aspects of emotional appraisal, including the amygdala (which is implicated in the detection and encoding of affectively arousing stimuli) and the insula (which receives viscerosensory inputs and appears to play a general role in affective experience).

Interestingly, reappraisal and suppression (the latter of which is often a maladaptive strategy) show interesting differences in brain activation. For suppression, late frontal engagement produced increasing amygdala–insula activity over time, whereas for reappraisal, early frontal engagement produced decreased amygdala–insula activity over time. This is consistent with findings showing that reappraisal and suppression, two regulation strategies with different effects on behavior, may depend upon similar control systems, albeit at different times (Ochsner & Gross, 2008).

My colleagues and I have presented a theoretical framework showing how anxious cognitions leading to avoidance are specifically a product of neural mechanisms of hyperreactivity (Hofmann, Ellard, & Siegle, 2012). According to this model, anxious cognitions are understood as decision points during the processing of threat information. After a potential threat is perceived and detected, subsequent decision points involve selecting adequate coping strategies and then applying those coping strategies with the goal of protecting oneself from threat and regulating the negative affect associated with the processing of threat. These decision points are associated with the activation of specific brain structures, depending on the level of information processing. The amygdala is involved at the early stage, followed by the hippocampus and the insular cortex, and later the anterior cingulate and prefrontal cortices (see Figure 8.1.).

Figure 8.1 shows that different brain structures are active at different points along the temporal dimension when emotions are elicited and experienced (see Chapter 1 for an in-depth discussion about the nature of emotions). It further distinguishes between the psychological, the biological, and the psychophysiological levels of emotional processing. This is not to suggest a cause-and-effect relationship of brain activation and emotional processing. Rather, it suggests an association between these levels, depending on the processing level of an emotion. Some pathological states, such as depression, seem to be associated with decreased prefrontal function, yielding

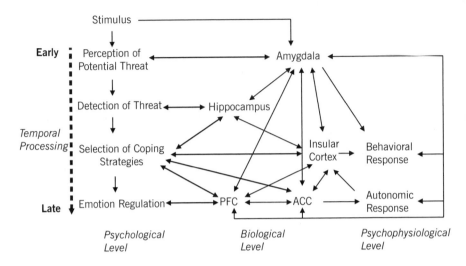

FIGURE 8.1. A cognitive–neurobiological model of fear and anxiety. From Hofmann, Ellard, and Siegle (2012). Copyright 2012 by Taylor & Francis. Reprinted by permission.

decreased regulatory control. Other emotional states, such as excessive fear and abnormal anxiety, involve preserved regulatory control in the presence of learned beliefs regarding the appropriateness and utility of avoidant coping strategies. Using such strategies can lead to the maintenance of these maladaptive emotional states (Hofmann, Ellard, et al., 2012).

The relationship between cognition and emotion and its brain correlates is intrinsically connected with the concept of the *default network* in brain sciences (Raichle, 2006). Since the emergence of modern brain sciences, two rivaling perspectives on brain functions have emerged. One perspective views the brain as a primarily reflexive organ, driven by the momentary demands of the environment; the other considers brain operations as mainly intrinsic in nature. Although the former perspective has been the dominant view in neuroscience research, accumulating evidence suggests that brain activity is not simply a response to external stimuli. Instead, it appears that when a person is awake and alert yet not actively engaged in an attention-demanding task, a default state of brain activity exists (Raichle et al., 2001; Raichle, 2006). Among other areas, this default state involves the medial PFC, the posterior cingulate, and precuneus. When focused attention is required (e.g., when novel information is presented), activity within these areas is attenuated, which reflects a necessary reduction in resources devoted to general information gathering and evaluation. In other words, it is believed that neurons continuously receive both excitatory inputs (i.e., information that tends to increase arousal) and inhibitory inputs (i.e., information that tends to decrease arousal). This "balance" might then be responsible for the brain's intrinsic activity that enables it to maintain and interpret information, as well as to respond to and possibly predict events in the environment. This principle applies to any brain activities, including those involved in emotions.

CORRELATES OF EMPATHY

It has been assumed that observing and imagining another person in a particular state activates a similar state in the observer. Observing or imagining another person's emotional state activates the same parts of the neurocircuitry that are involved in processing that same state in oneself (Preston & DeWaal, 2002). This is also known as the *perception–action model of empathy states*. Brain imaging studies have shown that this process is primarily associated with activation in the insula and the ACC (Ruby & Decety, 2004; Lutz, Brefczynski-Lewis, Johnstone, & Davidson, 2008; Lutz et al., 2009). Some of these studies examined brain activation using fMRI and psychophysiological correlates (heart rate) during meditation in Tibetan monks who had between 10,000 and 50,000 hours of meditation practice, much while performing LKM and CM (Lutz, Brefczynski-Lewis, et al., 2008; Lutz et al., 2009). In one of these studies, Lutz, Brefczynski-Lewis, and colleagues (2008) asked expert meditators and novices to either meditate or simply rest while they were presented with human vocalizations that were positive (baby laughing), neutral (background noise in a restaurant), or negative (distressed woman). Results showed that during meditation, activation in the insula was greater during presentation of negative sounds than positive or neutral sounds in the expert relative to the novice meditators. Moreover, the degree of insula activation was associated with self-reported intensity of the meditation in both groups. An analysis of a subsample further revealed that the activation of the dorsal ACC was associated with meditation, especially among the expert meditators, and that the right middle insula showed a greater association with heart rate across participants. This association was stronger in the left middle insula when experts were compared with novices (Lutz et al., 2009).

The insula is important in detecting emotions, in mapping physiological symptoms to emotions (such as heart rate), and in making this information available to other parts of the brain. Meditation appears to increase activity in the amygdala, which is important for the processing of emotional stimuli, and in the right temporal parietal juncture, an area that is implicated in empathy and when perceiving mental and emotional states of others. These studies suggest that LKM and CM may enhance the activation of brain areas that are involved in emotional processing and empathy.

A study by Pace and colleagues (2009) randomized healthy adults to 6 weeks of CM training or health discussions as a control condition and measured plasma cortisol (a stress hormone), plasma concentration of interleukin-6 (a substance involved in the inflammation response and the immune system), and subjective anxiety response to a social stress test that involves a social performance task. Although the groups showed no difference in plasma cortisol or interleukin-6 concentration, increased meditation practice was associated with decreased stress-induced interleukin-6 and subjective reports of distress in the meditation group. These findings suggest that CM reduces stress-induced subjective distress and immune response. However, because the stress test was administered after, rather than before, CM training, it is possible that associations between CM practice time and outcome in the stress task might have been due to differences in participants' stress response rather than to the practice itself. In order to address this weakness, the authors conducted a follow-up study with the identical paradigm, except that the stress test was conducted prior to the training (Pace et al., 2010). This time, no association was found between the stress response and subsequent amount of CM training. The authors interpreted these findings to suggest that CM reduces subjective and physiological responses to psychosocial stress.

INDIVIDUAL DIFFERENCES IN NEUROBIOLOGY

As noted earlier, the amygdala seems to be particularly important for processing fear and anxiety. This brain structure has a high gamma-aminobutyric acid (GABA) receptor density, and infants born with a lower density are more vulnerable to developing problems with fear or anxiety. GABA is the primary inhibitory neurotransmitter to counterbalance an excitatory neurotransmitter (glutamate). A deficiency in GABA (low concentration or low receptor density) can produce neuronal hyperexcitability, leading to anxiety disorders (Lydiard, 2003). Similarly, variation in dopamine and serotonin release and receptor density contributes to cortical excitability that is linked to excessive anxiety (Auerbach et al., 1999).

Neuroscience research also suggests that the amount of serotonin in the brain is associated with the ways the amygdala functions. Serotonin suppresses neuronal excitability, and children with lower levels of brain serotonin tend to be more distressed. Serotonin activity in the synapse is partly influenced by the presence of the serotonin transporter molecule, which absorbs serotonin from the synapse. The gene that codes for this molecule exists in the form of two alleles, a short and a long allele, located in the promoter region of the gene (an allele is a variant of a gene). The short allele is called "short" because the gene of this chromosome region is shorter than the other, the long allele. The short allele appears to be the risk allele because it is associated with less effective transcription of the gene. Carriers of this allele produce fewer transporter molecules, and serotonin remains active for a longer time. As a result, the production of serotonin is being suppressed, leading to greater excitability of the amygdala (Pezawas et al., 2005). Therefore, carriers of the short allele show greater amygdala activation to fear-provoking stimuli than carriers of the long allele of the serotonin transporter gene (Hariri et al., 2002). More recent research suggests that combinations of alleles, rather than single alleles, are associated with specific temperamental types. For example, 1-year-olds with extreme levels of avoidant behavior to a stranger showed both the short allele of the serotonin transporter gene and the short allele of the 7-repeat polymorphism of the dopamine D4 receptor, whereas the least avoidant children possessed the two long forms of the serotonin transporter gene with the 7-repeat polymorphism (Lakatos et al., 2003).

It has been shown that early aversive experiences, such as acute stress, can lead to neuroanatomical changes that can permanently affect future behaviors. For example, early experiences can affect the functioning of the limbic–hypothalamic–pituitary–adrenal system, as well as the GABA and benzodiazepine receptor systems (e.g., Anisman, Zaharia, Meany, & Merali, 1998; Caldji, Francis, Sharma, Plotzky, & Meany, 2000; Cicchetti & Rogosch, 2001). The time of the stressor determines the behavioral and cognitive consequences (Kolb, Gibb, & Gorny, 2001). Generally speaking, the earlier the insult, the greater the potential for neuroplasticity to compensate for any damages. However, the environment, including the person's culture, family, and relationship to the primary caregiver, among many other factors, are also important contributors (e.g., Olson & Sameroff, 2009).

CONCLUSION

The cognitive and affective neuroscience literature suggests that changes in emotions are directly associated with electrochemical changes in the brain. Important neurobiological correlates of emotions include the amygdala, the ventral and dorsal portions of the PFC, the dorsal portions of the ACC, the dorsal portions of the medial PFC, and the insula.

In the case of fear and anxiety, emotions are associated with early hyperreactivity and later recruitment of prefrontal resources associated with coping processes. Understanding these processes on the biological level can open up new windows of opportunities for research in the future, including new treatment targets.

This chapter exemplifies both the promise and the complexity of bridging emotion research and clinical science. By moving beyond the illness level of the latent medical disease model, we can begin a truly transdiagnostic and cross-disciplinary approach by studying emotions in clinical settings from a biological, neuropsychological, social, and motivational perspective. These different perspectives have the potential to significantly enhance our therapeutic methods to relieve our patients' suffering and enhance their quality of life and happiness.

Summary of Clinically Relevant Points

- Traditionally, laboratory experiments on fear in rats have contributed to theories about the neurobiological correlates of emotions. More recently, human experiments have been conducted analyzing participants' brain activity while they viewed emotional stimuli under different instructions to cope with their emotions.

- Neurobiological correlates of emotions include the amygdala, the ventral and dorsal portions of the PFC, the dorsal portions of the ACC, the dorsal portions of the medial PFC, and the insula.

- Cognitions can be understood as decision points in certain brain circuitries during the processing of information. In the case of fear, the initial decision points are the perception and detection of threat in the amygdala, followed by selecting adequate coping strategies that involve the hippocampus and the insular cortex, and then applying those coping strategies with the goal of protecting oneself from threat and regulating the negative affect (which involves the anterior cingulate and prefrontal cortices).

- Very little research exists on individual differences in neurobiological correlates of emotions. The most researched phenomenon is the relationship between emotional problems and the short allele of the serotonin transporter gene. There is also evidence that early stress can affect the functioning of the limbic–hypothalamic–pituitary–adrenal system, as well as the GABA and benzodiazepine receptor systems.

APPENDIX I

◆

Common Self-Report Measures

MOOD SCALES

- *Beck Depression Inventory* (BDI; Beck, Ward, Mendelson, Mock, & Erbaugh, 1961) and its revision (BDI-II; Beck, Steer, & Brown, 1996). The BDI and BDI-II each contain 21 questions. Answers are scored on a scale of 0 to 3.

- *Positive and Negative Affect Scale* (PANAS, Watson et al., 1988). The PANAS is a 20-item questionnaire that is divided into two 10-item subscales measuring positive affect (PANAS-PA) and negative affect (PANAS-NA). The questionnaire can be used with multiple time frames, including present moment, present day, past few days, past few weeks, year, and general.

ALEXITHYMIA

- *Toronto Alexithymia Scale* (TAS-20; Bagby, Parker, & Taylor, 1994a, 1994b). The TAS-20 is a 20-item scale consisting of three subscales: the Difficulty Describing Feeling subscale (5 items), the Difficulty Identifying Feeling subscale (7 items), and the Externally-Oriented Thinking subscale (8 items). The latter subscale measures the tendency of the person to focus his or her attention externally.

EMOTIONAL INTELLIGENCE

• *Emotional Intelligence Scale* (Schutte et al., 1998). The Emotional Intelligence Scale is a 33-item self-report scale to measure emotional intelligence based on the conceptualization by Salovey and Mayer (1990).

• *Trait Meta Mood Scale* (Salovey et al., 1995). The Trait Meta Mood Scale measures aspects of emotional intelligence, including attention to feelings, clarity of feelings, and mood repair.

AFFECTIVE STYLE

• *Affective Style Questionnaire* (ASQ; Hofmann & Kashdan, 2010). The ASQ is a 20-item scale consisting of three subscales: *Concealing* (8 items), *Adjusting* (7 items), and *Tolerating* (5 items) *Affect*, which maps onto the three different affective styles described above. There is no total scale score.

• *Emotion Regulation Questionnaire* (ERQ; Gross & John, 2003). The ERQ is a 10-item scale measuring individual differences in expressive suppression and cognitive reappraisal.

• *Acceptance and Action Questionnaire–II* (AAQ-II; Bond et al., 2011). The AAQ-II is a 10-item scale measuring individual differences in the willingness to accept and work with private thoughts and feelings in the pursuit of valued goals (an aggregation of multiple facets).

• *Difficulties in Emotion Regulation Scale* (DERS: Gratz & Roemer, 2004). The 36-item DERS measures various ways in which people habitually find themselves unable to successfully regulate difficult, aversive emotional experiences.

RUMINATION AND WORRYING

• *Ruminative Responses Scale* (RRS; Treynor et al., 2003). The RRS is a 10-item self-report questionnaire that assesses the extent to which participants engage in neutrally focused introspection (i.e., reflection) and "moody pondering" (i.e., brooding).

• *Penn State Worry Questionnaire* (PSWQ; Meyer, Miller, Metzger, & Borkovec, 1990). The PSWQ is a 16-item self-report instrument measuring the general tendency toward excessive worrying, without reference to specific content.

◆

Progressive Muscle Relaxation

Body and mind are closely connected. Emotional distress often leads to muscle tension and physiological arousal (i.e., increased heart rate, respiration), and calming one's body can also calm one's mind. Therefore, muscle tension is a good initial target for interventions aimed at reducing the intensity of emotional distress, because reducing muscle tension can also lower emotional arousal.

A well-developed and -tested approach for relaxing muscle tension is progressive muscle relaxation (PMR). The PMR approach initially takes approximately 30 minutes. With more experience, it is possible to use a 1-step technique, which can be done at any time or place. The longer 30-minute version of PMR can be very useful at the end of the day for decreasing muscle tension.

PMR comprises a set of simple instructions aimed at relaxing your muscles. As part of the instructions, the patient is asked to tense and release specific muscle groups. This teaches the client the distinction between feelings of muscle tension and of relaxation. Through PMR, people learn how to decrease the intensity of physiological arousal, and this, in turn, should also decrease the intensity of their emotion in general. It is important to remember that relaxation is a skill that requires repeated practice, just like learning how to ride a bike.

PMR starts with 12 muscle groups. Once clients have mastered the 12-muscle-group PMR, they are instructed to shift to the 8-muscle-group PMR. Clients are advised to practice PMR initially in nondistracting situations. Later, they may practice it in busier situations over time so that they become adept at relaxing anywhere, anytime. The basic instructions include the following:

1. *Close your eyes and take a few slow and normal breaths with your diaphragm (belly).*

2. *Tighten the muscles in both of your lower arms by making fists and pulling up on your wrists. Hold the tension for about 10 seconds. Now, relax these muscles and notice the difference between tension and relaxation (20 seconds).*

3. *Tighten your muscles in your upper arms by pulling your arms back and in to the sides of your body. Hold the tension for about 10 seconds. Now, relax these muscles and notice the difference between tension and relaxation (20 seconds).*

4. *Tighten your muscles in your lower legs by flexing your feet up and bringing your toes toward your upper body. Hold the tension for about 10 seconds. Now, relax these muscles and notice the difference between tension and relaxation (20 seconds).*

5. *Tighten your upper legs by bringing your knees together and lifting your legs off the chair. Hold the tension for about 10 seconds. Now, relax these muscles and notice the difference between tension and relaxation (20 seconds).*

6. *Tighten your stomach by pulling your stomach tightly in toward your spine. Hold the tension for about 10 seconds. Now, relax these muscles and notice the difference between tension and relaxation (20 seconds).*

7. *Tighten your chest by taking a deep breath and holding it. Hold the tension for about 10 seconds. Now, relax these muscles and notice the difference between tension and relaxation (20 seconds).*

8. *Tighten your shoulders by pulling them up toward your ears. Hold the tension for about 10 seconds. Now, relax these muscles and notice the difference between tension and relaxation (20 seconds).*

9. *Tighten your back of the neck by pushing your head back. Hold*

the tension for about 10 seconds. Now, relax these muscles and notice the difference between tension and relaxation (20 seconds).

10. *Purse your lips without clenching your teeth. Hold the tension for about 10 seconds. Now, relax these muscles and notice the difference between tension and relaxation (20 seconds).*

11. *Squint, so that your eyes are partly closed. Hold the tension for about 10 seconds. Now, relax these muscles and notice the difference between tension and relaxation (20 seconds).*

12. *Push your eyebrows together. Hold the tension for about 10 seconds. Now, relax these muscles and notice the difference between tension and relaxation (20 seconds). Tighten your upper forehead by raising up your eyebrows to the top of your head. Hold the tension for about 10 seconds. Now, relax these muscles and notice the difference between tension and relaxation (20 seconds).*

13. *Count in your mind slowly from one to five, making yourself feel more and more relaxed with every count. One: all of the tension is leaving your body. Two: you are dropping further and further down into relaxation. Three: you are feeling more and more relaxed. Four: you are completely relaxed. Five: embrace the feeling of complete relaxation. Feel the cool air as you breathe in and the warm air as you breathe out. Your breathing is slow and you are breathing normally with your belly. Every time you inhale, think of the word "relax" (2 minutes).*

14. *Now, count backward slowly from five and become more and more alert. Five–four–three–two–one, please open your eyes.*

Relaxation requires practice. People will differ in how well they can relax. Most people will have to practice the 12-muscle-group PMR daily for a few weeks. Once the patient is able to relax pretty well using the 12-muscle-group PMR, the therapist can introduce the PMR with only 8 muscle groups. The goal is to be able to achieve a relaxation state with just one step. The 8-muscle-group PMR focuses on the following areas:

1. *Both of your arms, with your lower and upper arms together*

2. *Both of your legs, with your lower and upper legs together*

3. *Your stomach*

4. *Your chest*

5. *Both of your shoulders*

6. *Your neck*

7. *Your eyes, and*

8. *Your upper and lower forehead together*

The sequence and pace is very similar to the 12-muscle-group PMR. Make sure that you concentrate on the difference between the tension and relaxation. Most people will need to practice the 8-muscle-group PMR daily for weeks until the effect is noticeable.

◆

Expressive Writing

The following case example discusses Peter, a man I treated for many months. To protect his privacy, I have changed key elements of his personal information.

In Practice: Writing about Emotions

Peter was a 35-year-old computer programmer who had been struggling with severe depression. In addition to major depressive disorder and dysthymia, he also met criteria for adult Asperger disorder. Interpersonally, he appeared awkward. For example, he spoke quickly, and his speech was difficult to understand. He did not pay much attention to his appearance. He often appeared at the sessions disheveled, his clothes were sometimes dirty, and his teeth were yellow and stained because of poor hygiene. His intelligence was clearly above normal, but he was awkward in social interactions. For example, he had a slight grin on his face, even when discussing sad, upsetting, and even traumatic events. Peter had a small circle of friends. He described a generally normal upbringing by his parents. However, he decided to discontinue a parent–son relationship with them when he began college. He reported that he broke off the relationship with his parents because they did not protect him when he was bullied in high school.

He reported that he had been severely and daily bullied by a number of children in his school. For example, one particular student, Bruce, would come up to him every morning at around the same time to punch him very hard in his stomach. On other occasions, Peter needed stitches for cuts from a knife and to remove a piece of pencil from his shoulder that another student, Jack, had stabbed him with. On yet another occasion, a girl named Lisa dragged him into the girl's bathroom to beat him up.

Although Peter was a good student, his teachers repeatedly recommended to his parents that he be moved to a different school because they could not ensure his safety or prevent the bullying. However, his father insisted that Peter should remain in school in order to "toughen up." Peter experienced high school as "hell." He had no friends who might have protected him from the bullies. His response to the attacks at school was to emotionally withdraw and to let the daily abuse happen without fighting back.

When Peter started college, he made friends with three other male students, and they formed a close circle. Despite his odd appearance and behavior, these friends accepted him and appreciated his intelligence and wit. Even after college, the bonds between Peter and especially two of his friends remained strong. Peter adopted them as his family. Although his friends felt uncomfortable with their roles and responsibilities in Peter's life, they continued to remain close friends, even after they married and had children. Peter expressed no sexual interest in women or men and did not want any children. After many years living alone during the week and spending most of his weekends with his friends, Peter moved in with one of his friends and took part in that friend's regular family activities. He paid a portion of the mortgage and cooked for the family most evenings (he had taken cooking classes in preparation for this living arrangement). His goal and desire was to be with his friends.

Peter expressed beliefs that bordered on delusional thinking. Specifically, he wanted to become a rich and powerful man. That would allow him to establish a society in which he could ban any violence so that nobody would have to experience the abuse he had been forced to endure. He had specific plans for how to build this society: He would become rich with a startup company (richer and more influential than Bill Gates). He would then establish a meritocracy in which people were judged and compensated solely based on their merits to society. However, he encountered many obstacles to implementing this plan, which led to a great deal of frustration and depression. Although he was a gifted and sought-out programmer, he always occupied a mediocre status in companies he worked for. He believed his depression was a direct consequence of these obstacles.

During treatment, it became clear that traditional strategies to target his depression, such as identifying and challenging maladaptive beliefs and enhancing behavioral activation, had little, if any, benefit. Moreover, targeting his grandiose beliefs about creating a meritocracy to improve the world was not successful when using traditional cognitive restructuring. In order to encourage the processing of some of his emotions, Peter was asked to describe a particular scene he encountered with his old schoolmate Jack. He wrote:

> I was hanging around the front of the school during recess, in 3rd grade, when Jack jabbed a pencil into my shoulder. Not much pain, lots of blood, and I was very much in shock. He was laughing and smiling. The pavement was hot and black, and a lot of other school kids were staring, a large percentage laughing and smiling. I told myself I was better than these jerks, and calmed myself. For the remainder of recess (perhaps 15 minutes), I went to class forgetting about my injury for a bit (maybe an additional 15 minutes) when I noticed the blood again. I informed the teacher I was injured and she gave me a pass for the nurse. Notably, she didn't ask how it happened, and while I didn't want to invite retribution, I was still surprised.

On another occasion, he wrote:

> I was perhaps in 5th grade, and during recess I was sitting around on the grass to the right side of the school when I was threatened by Jack holding a small knife. Looking back (many years later) I think he was trying to scare and bully me. I grabbed the knife by the blade, cutting my fingers quite badly. At the time, I was thinking this guy wants to kill me and either I stop him, or I die. I ran toward the school entrance where the teachers were. I then went to the nurse, and she called my mother to have her give me a ride to the hospital (judging the wounds to be minor). The assistant principal came in and asked me if I had instigated the fight (as that was what Jack was claiming). I said no, feeling indignant. The hospital, after having me put my hand in a bowl of water for a bit, judged the wounds more severe, leading me to believe the school nurse didn't care. And I got nine stitches. The next day, I found out Jack had been suspended, but he was back soon, and this was when Bruce, a guy in Jack's clique, started punching me in the gut daily. Good guys have it tough, I was thinking, as well as the world sucks.

Peter was asked to write a letter to Jack (not meant to be sent to him). Peter produced the following:

> Hi, Jack,
>
> It's Peter from [NAME OF SCHOOL]. I am writing today to get some things off my chest. Let me say first off that I understand that you were a kid

*tormented by your own demons, like most bullies, and I hope you have
turned your life around.*

*I was an odd, unpopular person in school as well as being physically
weak. So I comprehend, to an extent, why I was your target. . . .*

On another occasion, Peter wrote the following:

Dear Jack,

*Still a bad taste in my mouth from my experiences with you growing up.
That said, I have no interest in hating you as it only harms myself. I hope
you have changed, and want you to know that I unconditionally forgive
you for what you did to me, and with compassion upon you. I am torn only
because I do not believe you can change. I hope you can prove me wrong.*

Sincerely, Peter

These writing examples not only clarified the emotional struggles
the bullying episodes had caused the patient but they also led to emotional processing, resulting in significant improvements during treatment. Anger was replaced with forgiveness and even compassion for the
bully. This enabled Peter to resolve some of the trauma caused by these
early experiences that led to maladaptive beliefs and behaviors decades
later.

This was not an easy or quick process. Peter was seen for more than
2 years. Traditional cognitive-behavioral interventions were only moderately successful in improving his mood. The greatest gains in treatment
were seen after the loving-kindness meditation practices that included
images of Jack and other bullies in the meditation exercises. (I discuss
these practices in Chapter 7.) Peter eventually terminated treatment
because he felt he had reached a level of happiness sufficient for him to
continue his healing without further counseling.

References

Abramson, L. Y., & Seligman, M. E. (1978). Learned helplessness in humans: Critique and reformulation. *Journal of Abnormal Psychology, 87,* 49–74.

Ainsworth, M. D. S., Blehar, M. C., Waters, E., & Wall, S. (1978). *Patterns of attachment: A psychological study of the Strange Situation.* Hillsdale, NJ: Erlbaum.

Aldao, A., & Dixon-Gordon, K. L. (2014). Broadening the scope of research on emotion regulation strategies and psychopathology. *Cognitive Behaviour Therapy, 43,* 22–33.

Aldao, A., & Nolen-Hoeksema, S. (2012). When are adaptive strategies most predictive of psychopathology? *Journal of Abnormal Psychology, 121,* 276–281.

Aldao, A., Nolen-Hoeksema, S., & Schweizer, S. (2010). Emotion-regulation strategies across psychopathology: A meta-analytic review. *Clinical Psychology Review, 30,* 217–237.

Alloy, L. B., Abramson, L. Y., Tashman, N. A., Steinberg, D. L., Hogan, M. E., Whitehouse, W. G., et al. (2001). Developmental origins of cognitive vulnerability to depression: Parenting, cognitive, and inferential feedback styles of the parents of individuals at high and low cognitive risk for depression. *Cognitive Therapy and Research, 25,* 397–423.

Alloy, L. B., & Clements, C. M. (1992). Illusion of control: Invulnerability to negative affect and depressive symptoms after laboratory and natural stressors. *Journal of Abnormal Psychology, 101,* 234–245.

Allport, G .W. (1955). *Becoming.* New Haven, CT: Yale University Press.

American Psychiatric Association. (2013). *Diagnostic and statistical manual of mental disorders* (5th ed.). Arlington, VA: Author.

Amstadter, A. (2008). Emotion regulation and anxiety disorders. *Journal of Anxiety Disorders, 22,* 211–221.

Anālayo. (2003). *Satipatthana: The direct path to realization.* Birmingham, UK: Windhorse.

Anisman, H., Zaharia, M. D., Meany, M. J., & Merali, Z. (1998). Do early-life events permanently alter behavioral and hormonal responses to stressors? *International Journal of Developmental Neuroscience, 16,* 149–164.

Arch, J. J., & Craske, M. G. (2010). Laboratory stressors in clinically anxious and non-anxious individuals: The moderating role of mindfulness. *Behaviour Research and Therapy, 48,* 495–505.

Asnaani, A., Sawyer, A. T., Aderka, I. M., & Hofmann, S. G. (2013). Effect of suppression, reappraisal, and acceptance of emotional pictures on acoustic eye-blink startle magnitude. *Journal of Experimental Psychopathology, 4,* 182–193.

Auerbach, J., Geller, V., Lezer, S., Shinwell, E., Belmaker, R. H., & Levin, J. (1999) Dopamine D4 receptor (D4DR) and serotonin transporter promoter (5-HTTLPR) polymorphisms in the determination of temperament in 2-month-old infants. *Molecular Psychiatry, 4,* 369–373.

Bagby, R. M., Parker, J. D. A., & Taylor, G. J. (1994a). The Twenty-Item Toronto Alexithymia Scale—I: Item selection and crossvalidation of the factor structure. *Journal of Psychosomatic Research, 38,* 23–32.

Bagby, R. M., Parker, J. D. A., & Taylor, G. J. (1994b). The Twenty-Item Toronto Alexithymia Scale—II: Convergent, discriminant, and concurrent validity. *Journal of Psychosomatic Research, 38,* 33–40.

Bard, P. (1934). The neuro-humoral basis of emotional reactions. In C. Murchinson (Ed.), *Handbook of general experimental psychology* (pp. 264–311). Worcester, MA: Clark University Press.

Bargh, J. A., & Ferguson, M. J. (2000). Beyond behaviorism: On the automaticity of higher mental processes. *Psychological Review, 126,* 925–945.

Barlow, D. H. (2000). Unraveling the mysteries of anxiety and its disorders from the perspective of emotion therapy. *American Psychologist, 55,* 1247–1263.

Barlow, D. H. (2002). *Anxiety and its disorders: The nature and treatment of anxiety and panic* (2nd ed.). New York: Guilford Press.

Barlow, D. H., Allen. L. B., & Choate, M. L. (2004). Toward a unified treatment for emotional disorders. *Behavior Therapy, 35,* 205–230.

Barlow, D. H., Ellard, K. K., Sauer-Zvala, S., Bullis, J. R., & Carl, J. R. (2014). The origins of neuroticism. *Perspectives on Psychological Science, 9,* 481–496.

Barlow, D. H., Farchione, T. J., Fairholm, C. P., Elard, K. K., Boisseau, C. I., Allen, L. A., et al. (2010). *Unified protocol for transdiagnostic treatment of emotional disorders (therapist guide).* New York: Oxford University Press.

Barrett, L. F. (2004). Feelings or words?: Understanding the content in self-report ratings of experienced emotion. *Journal of Personality and Social Psychology, 87,* 266–281.

Barrett, L. F. (2014). Conceptual act theory: A precis. *Emotion Review, 6,* 292–297.

Barrett, L. F., Mesquita, B., Ochsner, K. N., & Gross, J. J. (2007). The experience of emotion. *Annual Review of Psychology, 58,* 373–403.

Baumeister, R. (2015). Conquer yourself, conquer the world. *Scientific American, 312,* 60–65.

Beck, A. T. (1979). *Cognitive therapy and the emotional disorders.* New York: New American Library/Meridian.

Beck, A. T. (2008). The evolution of the cognitive model of depression and its neurobiological correlates. *American Journal of Psychiatry, 165,* 969–977.

Beck, A. T., Steer, R. A., & Brown, G. K. (1996). *Manual for the Beck Depression Inventory–II.* San Antonio, TX: Psychological Corporation.

Beck. A. T., Ward, C. H., Mendelson, M., Mock, J., & Erbaugh, J. (1961). An inventory for measuring depression. *Archives of General Psychiatry, 4,* 561–571.

Bem, D. J. (1967). Self-perception: An alternative interpretation of cognitive dissonance phenomena. *Psychological Review, 74,* 183–200.

Bentham, J. (1988). *The principles of morals and legislation.* Amherst, NY: Prometheus Books. (Original work published 1789)

Berking, M. (2010). *Training emotionaler Kompetenzen* (2nd ed.). Berlin: Springer.

Berking, M., Ebert, D., Cuijpers, P., & Hofmann, S. G. (2013). Emotion regulation skills training enhances the efficacy of impatient cognitive behavioral therapy for major depressive disorder: A randomized controlled trial. *Psychotherapy and Psychosomatics, 82,* 234–245.

Berking, M., Margraf, M., Ebert, D., Wupperman, P., Hofmann, S. G., & Junghanns, K. (2011). Deficits in emotion-regulation skills predict alcohol use during and after cognitive behavioral therapy for alcohol dependence. *Journal of Consulting and Clinical Psychology, 79,* 307–318.

Berking, M., Wirtz, C. M., Svaldi, J., & Hofmann, S. G. (2014). Emotion regulation predicts symptoms of depression over five years. *Behaviour Research and Therapy, 57,* 13–20.

Berridge, K. C., Robinson, T. E., & Aldridge, J. W. (2009). Dissecting components of reward: 'Liking,' 'wanting,' and learning. *Current Opinion in Pharmacology, 9,* 65–73.

Bindra, D. (1974). A motivational view of learning, performance, and behavior modification. *Psychological Review, 81,* 199–213.

Bishop, M., Lau, S., Shapiro, L., Carlson, N. D., Anderson, J., Carmody Segal, Z. V., et al. (2004). Mindfulness: A proposed operational definition. *Clinical Psychology: Science and Practice, 11,* 230–241.

Bogg, T., & Roberts, B. W. (2004). Conscientiousness and health behaviors: A meta-analysis. *Psychological Bulletin, 130,* 887–919.

Bolles, R. C. (1972). Reinforcement, expectancy, and learning. *Psychological Review, 79*, 394–409.

Bonanno, G. A., & Burton, C. L. (2013). Regulatory flexibility: An individual differences perspective on coping and emotion regulation. *Perspectives on Psychological Science, 8*, 591–612,

Bonanno, G. A., Papa, A., O'Neil, K., Westphal, M., & Coifman, K. (2004). The importance of being flexible: The ability to enhance and suppress emotional expression predicts long-term adjustment. *Psychological Science, 15*, 482–487.

Bond, F. W., Hayes, S. C., Baer, R. A., Carpenter, K. M., Orcutt, H. K., Waltz, T., et al. (2011). Preliminary psychometric properties of the Acceptance and Action Questionnaire–II: A revised measure of psychological flexibility and experiential acceptance. *Behavior Therapy, 42*, 676–688.

Borkovec, T. D., & Hu, S. (1990). The effect of worry on cardiovascular response to phobic imagery. *Behaviour Research and Therapy, 28*, 69–73.

Borkovec, T. D., Ray, W. J., & Stöber, J. (1998). Worry: A cognitive phenomenon intimately linked to affective, physiological, and interpersonal behavioral processes. *Cognitive Therapy and Research, 22*, 561–576.

Bouchard, T. J. (2004). Genetic influence on human psychological traits. *Current Directions in Psychological Science, 13*, 148–151.

Bouton, M. E., Mineka, S., & Barlow, D. H. (2001). A modern learning theory perspective on the etiology of panic disorder. *Psychological Review, 108*, 4–32.

Bowlby, J. (1973). *Attachment and loss: Vol. 2. Separation: Anxiety and anger.* New York: Basic Books.

Bowlby, J. (1982). *Attachment and loss: Vol. 1. Attachment* (2nd ed.). New York: Basic Books.

Bradburn, N. M. (1969). *The structure of psychological well-being.* Chicago: Alpine.

Brickman, P., & Campbell, D. T. (1971). Hedonic relativism and planning the good society. In M. H. Appley (Ed.), *Adaptation-level theory* (pp. 287–305). New York: Academic Press.

Brooks-Gunn, J., & Lewis, M. (1984). Development of early visual self-recognition. *Developmental Review, 4*, 215–239.

Brown, G. W., & Harris, T. (1978). *Social origins of depression: A study of psychological disorder in women.* New York: Free Press.

Brown, K. W., Weinstein, N., & Creswell, J. D. (2012). Trait mindfulness modulates neuroendocrine and affective responses to social evaluative threat. *Psychoneuroendocrinology, 37*, 2037–2041.

Brown, T. A. (2007). Temporal course and structural relationships among dimensions of temperament and DSM-IV anxiety and mood disorder constructs. *Journal of Abnormal Psychology, 116*, 313–328.

Brown, T. A., & Barlow, D. H. (2009). A proposal for a dimensional classification system based on the shared features of the DSM-IV anxiety and mood disorders: Implications for assessment and treatment. *Psychological Assessment, 21,* 256–271.

Buddhaghosa. (1975). *Path of purification.* Kandy, Sri Lanka: Buddhist Publication Society.

Buddharakkhita, A. (1995). *Metta: The philosophy and practice of universal love.* Kandy, Sri Lanka: Buddhist Publication Society.

Bullis, J. R., Boe, H.-J., Asnaani, A., & Hofmann, S. G. (2014). The benefits of being mindful: Trait mindfulness predicts less stress reactivity to suppression. *Journal of Behavior Therapy and Experimental Psychiatry, 45,* 57–66.

Burns, D. D. (1980). *Feeling good: The new mood therapy.* New York: HarperCollins.

Buss, D. M. (Ed.). (1999). *Evolutionary psychology: The new science of the mind.* Needham Heights, MA: Allyn & Bacon.

Byrne, R., & Whiten, A. (1985). Tactical deception of familiar individuals in baboons (*Papio ursimus*). *Animal Behavior, 333,* 669–673.

Cacioppo, J. T., & Berntson, G. C. (1999). The affect system: Architecture and operating characteristics. *Current Directions in Psychological Science, 8,* 133–137.

Cacioppo, J. T., & Gardner, W. L. (1999). Emotion. *Annual Review of Psychology, 50,* 191–214.

Cacioppo, J. T., & Hawkley, L. C. (2003). Social isolation and health, with an emphasis on underlying mechanisms. *Perspectives in Biology and Medicine, 46,* S39–S52.

Caldji, C., Francis, D., Sharma, S., Plotzky, P. M., & Meany, M. J. (2000). The effects of early reading environment on the development of $GABA_A$ and central benzodiazepine receptor levels and novelty-induced fearfulness in the rat. *Neuropsychopharmacology, 22,* 219–229.

Campbell-Sills, L., Barlow, D. H., Brown, T. A., & Hofmann, S. G. (2006a). Acceptability of negative emotion in anxiety and mood disorders. *Emotion, 6,* 587–595.

Campbell-Sills, L., Barlow, D. H., Brown, T. A., & Hofmann, S. G. (2006b). Effects of suppression and acceptance on emotional responses of individuals with anxiety and mood disorders. *Behaviour Research and Therapy, 44,* 1251–1263.

Cannon, W. B. (1927). The James–Lange theory of emotions: A critical examination and an alternative theory. *American Journal of Psychology, 39,* 106–124.

Carl, J. R., Soskin, D. P., Kerns, C., & Barlow, D. H. (2013). Positive emotion regulation in emotional disorders: A theoretical review. *Clinical Psychology Review, 33,* 343–360.

Carmody, J., & Baer, R. A. (2009). How long does a mindfulness-based stress reduction program need to be?: A review of class contact hours and effect sizes for psychological distress. *Journal of Clinical Psychology, 65,* 627–638.

Carnevale, P. J. D., & Isen, A. M. (1986). The influence of positive affect and visual access on the discovery of integrative solutions in bilateral negotiation. *Organizational Behavior and Human Decision Processes, 37,* 1–13.

Carson, J. W., Keefe, F. J., Lynch, T. R., Carson, K. M., Goli, V., Fras, A. M., et al. (2005). Loving-kindness meditation for chronic low back pain: Results from a pilot trial. *Journal of Holistic Nursing, 23,* 287–304.

Carver, C. S., & Scheier, M. F. (1998). *On the self-regulation of behavior.* New York: Cambridge University Press.

Caspi, A., Moffitt, T. W., Newman, D. L., & Silva, P. A. (1996). Behavioral observations at age 3 years predict adult psychiatric disorders: Longitudinal evidence from a birth cohort. *Archives of General Psychiatry, 53,* 1033–1039.

Cassidy, J. (1994). Emotion regulation: Influences of attachment relationships. *Monographs of the Society for Research in Child Development, 59,* 228–283.

Chalmers, L. (2007). *Buddha's teachings: Being the sutta nipata, or discourse collection.* London: Oxford University Press.

Cheng, C. (2001). Assessing coping flexibility in real-life and laboratory settings: A multimethod approach. *Journal of Personality and Social Psychology, 80,* 814–833.

Cheng, C. (2003). Cognitive and motivational processes underlying coping flexibility: A dual-process model. *Journal of Personality and Social Psychology, 84,* 425–438.

Chida, Y., & Steptoe, A. (2008). Positive psychological well-being and mortality: A quantitative systematic review of prospective observational studies. *Psychosomatic Medicine, 70,* 741–756.

Cicchetti, D., & Rogosch, F. A. (2001). The impact of child maltreatment and psychopathology on neuroendocrine functioning. *Development and Psychopathology, 13,* 783–804.

Cioffi, D., & Holloway, J. (1993). Delayed costs of suppressed pain. *Journal of Personality and Social Psychology, 64,* 274–282.

Cisler, J. M., Olatunji, B. O., Feldner, M. T., & Forsyth, J. P. (2010). Emotion regulation and the anxiety disorders: An integrative review. *Journal of Psychopathology and Behavioral Assessment, 32,* 68–82.

Clark, D. A., & Beck, A. T. (2010). Cognitive theory and therapy of anxiety and depression: Convergence with neurobiological findings. *Trends in Cognitive Science, 14,* 418–424.

Clark, L. A., & Watson, D. (1991). Tripartite model of anxiety and depression: Psychometric evidence and taxonomic implications. *Journal of Abnormal Psychology, 100,* 316–336.

Clark, L. A., Watson, D., & Mineka, S. (1994). Temperament, personality, and the mood and anxiety disorders. *Journal of Abnormal Psychology, 103,* 103–116.

Coan, J. A. (2010). Adult attachment and the brain. *Journal of Social and Personal Relationships, 27,* 210–217.

Coan, J. A. (2011). The social regulation of emotion. In J. Decety & J. T. Cacioppo (Eds.), *Handbook of social neuroscience* (pp. 614–623). New York: Oxford University Press.

Cohen, S. (2004). Social relationships and health. *American Psychologist, 59,* 676–684.

Cole, P. M., Martin, S. E., & Dennis, T. A. (2004). Emotion regulation as a scientific construct: Methodological challenges and directions for child development research. *Child Development, 75,* 317–333.

Colibazzi, T., Posner, J., Wang, Z., Gorman, D., Gerber, A., Yu, S., et al. (2010). Neural systems subserving valence and arousal during the experience of induced emotions. *Emotion, 10,* 377–389.

Compas, B. E., Malcarne, V., & Fondacaro, K. M. (1988). Coping with stressful events in older children and young adolescents. *Journal of Consulting and Clinical Psychology, 56,* 405–411.

Condon, P., Desbordes, G., Miller, W. B., & DeSteno, D. (2013). Meditation increases compassionate responses to suffering. *Psychological Science, 24,* 2125–2127.

Consedine, N., Magai, C., & Bonanno, G. A. (2002). Moderators of the emotion inhibition–health relationship: A review and research agenda. *Review of General Psychology, 6,* 204–238.

Cooley, C. H. (1902). *Human nature and the social order.* New York: Scribner's.

Cooper, R. K., & Sawaf, A. (1997). *Executive EQ: Emotional intelligence in leadership and organizations.* New York: Grosset/Putnam.

Cox, W. M., & Klinger, E. (1988). A motivational model of alcohol use. *Journal of Abnormal Psychology, 97,* 168–180.

Craig, W. (1918). Appetites and aversions as constituents of instincts. *Biological Bulletin of Woods Hole, 34,* 91–107.

Craske, M. G. (1999). *Anxiety disorders. Psychological approaches to theory and treatment.* Boulder, CO: Westview Press.

Dalai Lama. (2001). *An open heart: Practicing compassion in everyday life.* Boston: Little, Brown.

Dalai Lama, & Cutler, H. C. (1998). *The art of happiness: A handbook for living.* New York: Riverhead Books.

Darwin, C. (1955). *Expression of the emotions in man and animals.* New York: Philosophical Library. (Original work published 1872)

Davey, G. C. L. (1994). Worrying, social problem-solving abilities, and social problem-solving confidence. *Behaviour Research and Therapy, 32,* 327–330.

Davey, G. C. L., Jubb, M., & Cameron, C. (1996). Catastrophic worrying as a function of changes in problem-solving confidence. *Cognitive Therapy and Research, 20,* 333–344.

Davidson, R. J. (2003). Darwin and the neural bases of emotion and affective style. *Proceedings of the New York Academy of Sciences, 1000,* 316–336.

Davidson, R. J., & Begley, S. (2012). *The emotional life of your brain: How its unique patterns affect the way you think, feel, and live—and how you can change them*. New York: Hudson Street Press.

Davidson, R. J., Jackson, D. C., & Kalin, N. H. (2000). Emotion, plasticity, context, and regulation: Perspectives from affective neuroscience. *Psychological Bulletin, 126*, 890–909.

Davis, M., & Whalen, P. J. (2001). The amygdala: Vigilance and emotion. *Molecular Psychiatry, 6*, 13–34.

DeNeve, K. M., & Cooper, H. (1998). The happy personality: A meta-analysis of 137 personality traits and subjective well-being. *Psychological Bulletin, 124*, 197–229.

Derryberry, D., & Rothbart, M. K. (1997). Reactive and effortful processes in the organization of temperament. *Development and Psychopathology, 9*, 633–652.

DeRubeis, R. J., Siegle, G. J., & Hollon, S. D. (2008). Cognitive therapy versus medication for depression: Treatment outcomes and neural mechanisms. *Nature Review Neuroscience, 9*, 788–796.

de Waal, F. (1982). *Chimpanzee politics: Power and sex among apes*. New York: Harper & Row.

Diener, E. (2000). Subjective well-being: The science of happiness and a proposal for a national index. *American Psychologist, 55*, 34–43.

Diener, E., & Diener, M. (1995). Cross-cultural correlates of life satisfaction and self-esteem. *Journal of Personality and Social Psychology, 68*, 653–663.

Diener, E., & Seligman, M. E. P. (2002). Very happy people. *Psychological Science, 13*, 81–84.

Duval, S., & Wicklund, R. (1972). *A theory of objective self-awareness*. New York: Academic Press.

Ehrenreich, J. T., Fairholm, C. P., Buzzella, B. A., Ellard, K. K., & Barlow, D. H. (2007). The role of emotion in psychological therapy. *Clinical Psychology: Science and Practice, 14*, 422–428.

Eisenberg, N., Spinrad, T. L., & Eggum, N. D. (2010). Emotion-related self-regulation and its relation to children's maladjustment. *Annual Review of Clinical Psychology, 6*, 495–525.

Ekman, P. (1992a). An argument for basic emotions. *Cognition and Emotion, 6*, 169–200.

Ekman, P. (1992b). Are there basic emotions? *Psychological Review, 99*, 550–553.

Ekman, P. (2003). *Emotions revealed*. New York: Times Books.

Ekman, P., Friesen, W. V., & Ellsworth, P. (1972). *Emotion in the human face: Guidelines for research and an integration of findings*. New York: Plenum Press.

Ellis, A. (1962). *Reason and emotion in psychotherapy*. New York: Lyle Stuart.

Emmons, R. A. (1986). Personal strivings: An approach to personality and subjective well-being. *Journal of Personality and Social Psychology, 51,* 1058–1068.

Epictetus. (2013). *The Enchiridion of Epictetus.* New York: Start Publishing. (Original work published 135 C.E.)

Epstein, R. P. (2006). The molecular genetic architecture of human personality: Beyond self-report questionnaires. *Molecular Psychiatry, 11,* 427–445.

Epstude, K., & Roese, N. J. (2008). The functional theory of counterfactual thinking. *Personality and Social Psychology Review, 12,* 168–192.

Estrada, C. A., Isen, A. M., & Young, M. J. (1997). Positive affect facilitates integration of information and decreases anchoring in reasoning among physicians. *Organizational Behavior and Human Decision Processes, 72,* 117–135.

Feldman, C. (2005). *Compassion.* Berkeley, CA: Rodnell Press.

Feldman, G., Dunn, E., Stemke, C., Bell, K., & Greeson, J. (2014). Mindfulness and rumination as predictors of persistence with a distress tolerance task. *Personality and Individual Differences, 56,* 154–158.

Feldman, L. A. (1995a). Valence focus and arousal focus: Individual differences in the structure of affective experience. *Journal of Personality and Social Psychology, 69,* 153–166.

Feldman, L. A. (1995b). Variations in the circumplex structure of mood. *Personality and Social Psychology Bulletin, 21,* 806–817.

Fenigstein, A., Scheier, M. F., & Buss, A. H. (1975). Public and private self-consciousness: Assessment and theory. *Journal of Consulting and Clinical Psychology, 43,* 522–527.

Festinger, L. (1954). A theory of social comparison processes. *Human Relations, 7,* 117–140.

Festinger, L., & Carlsmith, J. M. (1959). Cognitive consequences of forced compliance. *Journal of Abnormal and Social Psychology, 58,* 203–210.

Fincham, F. D., Beach, S. R., Harold, G. T., & Osborne, L. N. (1997). Marital satisfaction and depression: Different causal relationships for men and women? *Psychological Science, 8,* 351–357.

Flynn, M., & Rudolph, K.D. (2010). The contribution of deficits in emotional clarity to stress responses and depression. *Journal of Applied Developmental Psychology, 31,* 291–297.

Foa, E. B., & Kozak, M. J. (1986). Emotional processing of fear: Exposure to corrective information. *Psychological Bulletin, 99,* 20–35.

Folkman, S., & Moskowitz, J. T. (2004). Coping: Pitfalls and promise. *Annual Review of Psychology, 55,* 745–774.

Fowles, D. C. (1993). Biological variables in psychopathology: A psychobiological perspective. In P. B. Sutker & H. E. Adams (Eds.), *Comprehensive handbook of psychopathology* (2nd ed., pp. 57–82). New York: Plenum Press.

Fraley, R. C., & Shaver, P. R. (2000). Adult romantic attachment: Theoretical developments, emerging controversies, and unanswered questions. *Review of General Psychology, 4,* 132–154.

Fredrickson, B. L. (2000). What good are positive emotions? *Review of General Psychology, 2,* 300–319.

Fredrickson, B. L., & Branigan, C. (2005). Positive emotions broaden the scope of attention and thought–action repertoires. *Cognition and Emotion, 19,* 313–332.

Fredrickson, B. L., Cohn, M. A., Coffey, K. A., Pek, J., & Finkel, S. M. (2008). Open hearts build lives: Positive emotions, induced through loving-kindness meditation, build consequential personal resources. *Journal of Personality and Social Psychology, 95,* 1045–1061.

Fresco, D. M., Frankel, A. N., Mennin, D. S., Turk, C. L., & Heimberg, R. G. (2002). Distinct and overlapping features of rumination and worry: The relationship of cognitive production to negative affective states. *Cognitive Therapy and Research, 26,* 179–188.

Frijda, N. H. (1986). *The emotions.* Cambridge, UK: Cambridge University Press.

Frijda, N. H. (1988). The laws of emotion. *American Psychologist, 43,* 349–358.

Frydenberg, E. (1997). *Adolescent coping: Research and theoretical perspectives.* London: Routledge.

Gable, P. A., & Harmon-Jones, E. (2011). Attentional consequences of pregoal and postgoal positive affects. *Emotion, 11,* 1358–1367.

Gallup, G. G. (1970). Chimpanzees: Self-recognition. *Science, 167,* 86–87.

Gallup, G. G. (1979). Self-awareness in primates. *American Scientist, 67,* 417–421.

George, L. K., Blazer, D. G., Hughes, D. C., & Fowler, N. (1989). Social support and the outcome of major depression. *British Journal of Psychiatry, 154,* 478–485.

Gergen, K. J. (1971). *The concept of self.* New York: Holt, Rinehart & Winston.

Gilbert, D. (2006). *Stumbling on happiness.* New York: Alfred Knopf.

Gilbert, D., & Wilson, T. D. (2007). Prospection: Experiencing the future. *Science, 317,* 1351–1354.

Gilbert, P., & Procter, S. (2006). Compassionate mind training for people with high shame and self-criticism: Overview and pilot study of a group therapy approach. *Clinical Psychology and Psychotherapy, 13,* 353–379.

Gohm, C. L., & Clore, G. L. (2000). Individual differences in emotional experience: Mapping available scales to processes. *Personality and Social Psychology Bulletin, 26,* 679–697.

Goleman, D. (1995). *Emotional intelligence.* New York: Bantam Books.

Goodall, J. (1971). *In the shadow of man.* Boston: Houghton Mifflin.

Gratz, K. L., & Roemer, L. (2004). Multidimensional assessment of emotion regulation and dysregulation: Development, factor structure, and initial validation of the Difficulties in Emotion Regulation Scale. *Journal of Psychopathology and Behavioral Assessment, 26,* 41–54.

Gray, J. A. (1987). *The psychology of fear and stress.* Cambridge, UK: Cambridge University Press.

Gray, J. A. (1990). Brain systems that mediate emotion and cognition. *Cognition and Emotion, 4,* 269–288.

Gray, J. A., & McNaughton, N. (1996). The neuropsychology of anxiety: Reprise. In D. A. Hope (Ed.), *Nebraska Symposium on Motivation: Vol. 43. Perspectives on anxiety, panic, and fear* (pp. 61–134). Lincoln: University of Nebraska Press.

Gray, J. A., & McNaughton, N. (2000). *The neuropsychology of anxiety* (2nd ed.). Oxford, UK: Oxford University Press.

Greenberg, L. S. (2011). *Emotion-focused therapy.* Washington, DC: American Psychological Association.

Greenberg, L. S., & Paivio, S. C. (1997). *Working with emotions in psychotherapy.* New York: Guilford Press.

Greenberg, L. S., & Safran, J. D. (1987). *Emotion in psychotherapy.* New York: Guilford Press.

Gross, J. J. (1998a). Antecedent- and response-focused emotion regulation: Divergent consequences for experience, expression, and physiology. *Journal of Personality and Social Psychology, 74,* 224–237.

Gross, J. J. (1998b). The emerging field of emotion regulation: An integrative review. *Review of General Psychology, 2,* 271–299.

Gross, J. J. (2013). *Handbook of emotion regulation* (2nd ed.). New York: Guilford Press.

Gross, J. J., & John, O. P. (2003). Individual differences in two emotion regulation processes: Implications for affect, relationships, and well-being. *Journal of Personality and Social Psychology, 85,* 348–362.

Gross, J. J., & Levenson, R. W. (1997). Hiding feelings: The acute effects of inhibiting negative and positive emotion. *Journal of Abnormal Psychology, 106,* 95–103.

Grossman, P., Niemann, L., Schmidt, S., & Walach, H. (2004). Mindfulness-based stress reduction and health benefits: A meta-analysis. *Journal of Psychosomatic Research, 57,* 35–43.

Gruzelier, J. H. (1989). Lateralization and central mechanisms in clinical psychophysiology. In G. Turpin (Ed.), *Handbook of clinical psychophysiology* (pp. 135–174). New York: Wiley.

Haber, M. G., Cohen, J. L., Lucas, T., & Baltes, B. B. (2007). The relationship between self-reported received and perceived social support: A meta-analytic review. *American Journal of Community Psychology, 39,* 133–144.

Hamilton, W. D. (1964). The genetic evolution of social behavior. *Journal of Theoretical Biology, 7,* 1–52.

Hariri, A. R., Mattoy, B. S., Tessitore, A., Fera, F., Smith, W. T., & Weinberger, D. R. (2002). Extroamphetamine modulates the response of the human amygdala. *Neurosystems Pharmacology, 27,* 1036–1040.

Harmon-Jones, E., Harmon-Jones, C., & Price, T. F. (2013). What is approach motivation? *Emotion Review, 5,* 291–295.

Harris, C. R. (2001). Cardiovascular responses of embarrassment and effects of emotional suppression in a social setting. *Journal of Personality and Social Psychology, 81,* 886–897.

Harter, S. (1999). *The construction of the self: A developmental perspective.* New York: Guilford Press.

Hayes, S. C. (2004). Acceptance and commitment therapy, relational frame theory, and the third wave of behavior therapy. *Behavior Therapy, 35,* 639–665.

Hayes, S. C., Luoma, J., Bond, F., Masuda, A., & Lillis, J. (2006). Acceptance and commitment therapy: Model, processes, and outcomes. *Behaviour Research and Therapy, 44,* 1–25.

Hayes, S. C., Strosahl, K. D. , & Wilson, K. G. (1999). *Acceptance and commitment therapy: An experiential approach to behavior change.* New York: Guilford Press.

Heller, W., Nitschke, J. B., Etienne, M. A., & Miller, G. A. (1997). Patterns of regional brain activity differentiate types of anxiety. *Journal of Abnormal Psychology, 106,* 376–385.

Higgins, E. T. (1987). Self-discrepancy: A theory relating self and affect. *Psychological Review, 94,* 309–340.

Higgins, E. T., & Pittman, T. S. (2008). Motives of the human animal: Comprehending, managing, and sharing inner states. *Annual Review of Psychology, 59,* 361–385.

Hoehn-Saric, R., & McLeod, D. R. (2000). Anxiety and arousal: Physiological changes and their perception. *Journal of Affective Disorders, 61,* 217–224.

Hofer, M.A. (2006). Psychobiological roots of early attachment. *Current Directions in Psychological Science, 15,* 84–88.

Hofmann, S. G. (2000). Self-focused attention before and after treatment of social phobia. *Behaviour Research and Therapy, 38,* 717–725.

Hofmann, S. G. (2004). Cognitive mediation of treatment change in social phobia. *Journal of Consulting and Clinical Psychology, 72,* 392–399.

Hofmann, S. G. (2007). Cognitive factors that maintain social anxiety disorder: A comprehensive model and its treatment implications. *Cognitive Behaviour Therapy, 36,* 195–209.

Hofmann, S. G. (2008). Cognitive processes during fear acquisition and extinction in animals and humans: Implications for exposure therapy of anxiety disorders. *Clinical Psychology Review, 28,* 199–210.

Hofmann, S. G. (2011). *An introduction to modern CBT: Psychological solutions to mental health problems.* Oxford, UK: Wiley-Blackwell.

Hofmann, S. G. (2014). Interpersonal emotion regulation model of mood and anxiety disorders. *Cognitive Therapy and Research, 38,* 483–492.

Hofmann, S. G., Asmundson, G. J., & Beck, A. T. (2013). The science of cognitive therapy. *Behavior Therapy, 44,* 199–212.

Hofmann, S. G., Asnaani, A., Vonk, J. J., Sawyer, A. T., & Fang, A. (2012). The efficacy of cognitive behavioral therapy: A review of meta-analyses. *Cognitive Therapy and Research, 36,* 427–440.

Hofmann, S. G., Ellard, K., & Siegle, G. (2012). Neurobiological correlates of cognitions in fear and anxiety: A cognitive–neurobiological information-processing model. *Cognition and Emotion, 26,* 282–299.

Hofmann, S. G., Grossman, P., & Hinton, D. E. (2011). Loving-kindness and compassion meditation: Potential for psychological interventions. *Clinical Psychology Review, 31,* 1126–1132.

Hofmann, S. G., Heering, S., Sawyer, A. T., & Asnaani, A. (2009). How to handle anxiety: The effects of reappraisal, acceptance, and suppression strategies on anxious arousal. *Behaviour Research and Therapy, 47,* 380–394.

Hofmann, S. G., & Heinrichs, N. (2002). Disentangling self-descriptions and self-evaluations under conditions of high self-focused attention: Effects of mirror exposure. *Personality and Individual Differences, 32,* 611–620.

Hofmann, S. G., & Kashdan, T. B. (2010). The Affective Style Questionnaire: Development and psychometric properties. *Journal of Psychopathology and Behavioral Assessment, 32,* 255–263.

Hofmann, S. G., Moscovitch, D. A., Kim, H.-J., & Taylor, A. N. (2004). Changes in self-perception during treatment of social phobia. *Journal of Consulting and Clinical Psychology, 72,* 588–596.

Hofmann, S. G., Moscovitch, D. A., Litz, B. T., Kim, H.-J., Davis, L., & Pizzagalli, D. A. (2005). The worried mind: Autonomic and prefrontal activation during worrying. *Emotion, 5,* 464–475.

Hofmann, S. G., Sawyer, A. T., Fang, A., & Asnaani, A. (2012). Emotion dysregulation model of mood and anxiety disorders. *Depression and Anxiety, 29,* 409–416.

Hofmann, S. G., Sawyer, A. T., Witt, A., & Oh, D. (2010). The effect of mindfulness-based therapy on anxiety and depression: A meta-analytic review. *Journal of Consulting and Clinical Psychology, 78,* 169–183.

Hofstede, G. (1984). The cultural relativity of the quality of life concept. *Academy of Management Review, 9,* 389–398.

Hohmann, G. W. (1966). Some effects of spinal cord lesions on experienced emotional feelings. *Psychophysiology, 3,* 143–156.

Hollon, S. D., & Ponniah, K. (2010). A review of empirically supported psychological therapies for mood disorders in adults. *Depression and Anxiety, 27,* 891–932.

Hölzel, B., Lazar, S. W., Gard, T., Schuman-Olivier, Z., Vago, D. R., & Ott, U. (2011). How does mindfulness meditation work?: Proposing mechanisms of action from a conceptual and neural perspective. *Perspectives on Psychological Science, 6,* 537–559.

Hopkins, J. (2001). *Cultivating compassion.* New York: Broadway Books.

Hull, C. L. (1943). *Principles of behavior: An introduction to behavior therapy*. New York: Appleton-Century.

Humphrey, N. K. (1976). The social function of intellect. In P. P. G. Bateson & R. A. Hinde (Eds.), *Growing points in ethology* (pp. 303–317). Cambridge, UK: Cambridge University Press.

Hutcherson, C. A., Seppala, E. M., & Gross, J. J. (2008). Loving-kindness meditation increases social connectedness. *Emotion, 8*, 720–724.

Ingram, R. E. (1990). Self-focused attention in clinical disorders: Review and a conceptual modal. *Psychological Bulletin, 107*, 156–176.

Insel, T. R., & Collins, F. S. (2003). Psychiatry in the genomics era. *American Journal of Psychiatry, 160*, 616–620.

Izard, C. E. (1992). Basic emotions, relations among emotions, and emotion–cognition relations. *Psychological Review, 99*, 561–565.

James, W. W. (1884). What is emotion? *Mind, 4*, 188–204.

James, W. W. (1983). *Principles of psychology*. Cambridge, MA: Harvard University Press. (Original work published 1890)

Johnson, K. J., & Fredrickson, B. L. (2005). "We all look the same to me": Positive emotions eliminate the own-race bias in face recognitions. *Psychological Science, 16*, 875–881.

Johnson, S. L., & Jacob, T. (1997). Marital interactions of depressed men and women. *Journal of Consulting and Clinical Psychology, 65*, 15–23.

Joiner, T. (1997). Shyness and low social support as interactive diathesis, with loneliness as mediator: Testing an interpersonal-personality view of vulnerability to depressive symptoms. *Journal of Abnormal Psychology, 106*, 386–394.

Jolly, A. (1966). Lemur social intelligence and primate intelligence. *Science, 153*, 501–506.

Kabat-Zinn, J. (2003). Mindfulness-based interventions in context: Past, present, and future. *Clinical Psychology: Science and Practice, 10*, 144–156.

Kagan, J., & Snidman, N. (2004). *The long shadow of temperament*. Cambridge, MA: Harvard University Press.

Kahneman, D. (2011). *Thinking fast and slow*. New York: Farrar, Straus & Giroux.

Kahneman, D., Diener, E., & Schwarz, N. (2003). *Well-being: The foundations of hedonic psychology*. New York: Russell Sage Foundation.

Kashdan, T. B., & Rottenberg, J. (2010). Psychological flexibility as a fundamental aspect of health. *Clinical Psychology Review, 30*, 865–878.

Kendall, P. C., & Hollon, S. D. (1981). Assessing self-referent speech: Methods in the measurement of self-statements. In P. C. Kendall & S. D. Hollon (Eds.), *Assessment strategies for cognitive-behavioral interventions* (pp. 85–118). New York: Academic Press.

Kern, M. L., & & Friedman, H. S. (2008). Do conscientious individuals live longer?: A quantitative review. *Health Psychology, 27*, 505–512.

Khoury, B., Lecomte, T., Fortin, G., Masse, M., Therien, P., Bouchard, V., et al. (2013). Mindfulness-based therapy: A comprehensive meta-analysis. *Clinical Psychology Review, 33*, 763–771.

Killingsworth, M. A., & Gilbert, D. T. (2010). A wandering mind is an unhappy mind. *Science, 330*, 932.

Kircanski, K., Lieberman, M. D., & Craske, M. G. (2012). Feelings into words: Contributions of language to exposure therapy. *Psychological Science, 23*, 1086–1091.

Koenders, P. G., & van Strien, T. (2001) Emotional eating, rather than lifestyle behavior, drives weight gain in a prospective study in 1562 employees. *Journal of Occupational Environmental Medicine, 53*, 1287–1293.

Koivumaa-Honkanen, H., Honkanen, R., Viinamaeki, H., Heikkilae, K., Kaprio, J., & Koskenvuo, M. (2001). Life satisfaction and suicide: A 20-year follow-up study. *American Journal of Psychiatry, 158*, 433–439.

Kolb, B., Gibb, R., & Gorny, G. (2001). Cortical plasticity and the development of behavior after early frontal cortical injury. *Developmental Neuropsychology, 18*, 423–444.

Kring, A. M., Barrett, L. F., & Gard, D. E. (2003). On the broad applicability of the affective circumplex: Representations of affective knowledge among schizophrenia patients. *Psychological Science, 14*, 207–214.

Kringelbach, M. L., & Berridge, K. C. (2010). *Pleasures of the brain.* Oxford, UK: Oxford University Press.

Kristeller, J. L. (2007). Mindfulness meditation. In P. Lehrer, R. L. Woolfolk, & W. E. Sime (Eds.), *Principles and practice of stress management* (3rd ed., pp. 393–427). New York: Guilford Press.

Kubzansky, L. D., & Thurston, R. C. (2007). Emotional vitality and incident of coronary heart disease: Benefits of healthy psychological functioning. *Archives of General Psychiatry, 64*, 1393–1401.

Ladouceur, R., Gosslin, P., & Dugas, M. J. (2000). Experimental manipulation of intolerance of uncertainty: A study of a theoretical model of worry. *Behaviour Research and Therapy, 38*, 933–941.

Lakatos, K., Nemoda, Z., Birkas, E., Ronai, Z., Kovacs, E., Ney, K., et al. (2003). Association of D4 dopamine receptor gene and serotonin transporter promoter polymorphism with infants' response to novelty. *Molecular Psychiatry, 8*, 90–98.

Lakey, B., Orehek, E., Hain, K. L., & Van Vleet, M. (2010). Enacted support's links to negative affect and perceived support are more consistent with theory when social influences are isolated from trait influences. *Personality and Social Psychology Bulletin, 36*, 132–142.

Lang, P. J., Bradley, M. M., & Cuthbert, B. N. (1990). Emotion, attention, and the startle reflex. *Psychological Review, 97*, 377–395.

Lange, C. (1887). *Über Gemütsbewegungen [About emotions].* Leipzig, Germany.

Langer, E. J. (1989). *Mindfulness.* Reading, MA; Addison-Wesley.

Langer, E. J., & Moldoveanu, M. (2000). The construct of mindfulness. *Journal of Social Issues, 56*, 1–9.

Lazarus, R. S. (1966). *Psychological stress and the coping process.* New York: McGraw-Hill.

Lazarus, R. S. (1981). The stress and coping paradigm. In C. Eisdorfer, D. Cohen, A. Kleinman, & P. Maxim (Eds.), *Models for clinical psychopathology* (pp. 177–214). New York: Spectrum.

Lazarus, R. S. (1991). *Emotion and adaptation.* New York: Oxford University Press.

Lazarus, R. S. (2000). Toward better research on stress and coping. *American Psychologist, 55,* 665–673.

Lazarus, R. S., DeLongis, A., Folkman, S., & Gruen, R. (1985). Stress and adaptational outcomes: The problem of confounded measures. *American Psychologist, 40,* 770–779.

Lazarus, R. S., & Folkman, S. (1984). *Stress, appraisal, and coping.* New York: Springer.

Leahy, R. L., Tirch, D., & Napolitano, L. A. (2011). *Emotion regulation in psychotherapy: A practitioner's guide.* New York: Guilford Press.

Leary, M. R., Tate, E. B., Adams, C. E., Allen, A. B., & Hancock, J. (2007). Self-compassion and reactions to unpleasant self-relevant events: The implications of treating oneself kindly. *Journal of Personality and Social Psychology, 92,* 887–904.

LeDoux, J. E. (2000). Emotion circuits in the brain. *Annual Review of Neuroscience, 23,* 155–184.

LeDoux, J. E. (2015). *Anxious: Using the brain to understand and treat fear and anxiety.* New York: Viking.

Leyro, T., Zvolensky, M., & Bernstein, A. (2010). Distress tolerance and psychopathological symptoms and disorders: A review of the empirical literature among adults. *Psychological Bulletin, 136,* 576–600.

Lim, D., Condon, P., & DeSteno, D. (2015). Mindfulness and compassion: An examination of mechanism and scalability. *PLoS ONE, 10,* e0118221.

Lucas, R. E., Diener, E., & Grob, A. (2000). Cross-cultural evidence for the fundamental features of extraversion. *Journal of Personality and Social Psychology, 79,* 452–468.

Lucas, R. E., Diener, E., & Suh, E. M. (1996). Discriminant validity of well-being measures. *Journal of Personality and Social Psychology, 71,* 616–628.

Lunkenheimer, E. S., Shields, A. M., & Cortina, K. S. (2007). Parental emotion coaching and dismissing in family interaction. *Social Development, 16,* 232–248.

Lutz, A., Brefczynski-Lewis, J., Johnstone, T., & Davidson, R. J. (2008). Regulation of the neural circuitry of emotion by compassion meditation: Effects of meditative expertise. *PLoS ONE, 3,* e1897.

Lutz, A., Greischar, L., Perlman, D. M., & Davidson, R. J. (2009). BOLD signal in insula is differentially related to cardiac function during compassion meditation in experts vs. novices. *NeuroImage, 47,* 1038–1046.

Lutz, A., Slagter, H. A., Dunne, J. D., & Davidson, R. (2008). Attention regulation and monitoring and meditation. *Trends in Cognitive Sciences, 12,* 163–169.

Lydiard, R. B. (2003). The role of GABA in anxiety disorder. *Journal of Clinical Psychiatry, 64*(Suppl. 3), 21–27.

Lyonfields, J. D., Borkovec, T. D., & Thayer, J. F. (1995). Vagal tone in generalized anxiety disorder and the effects of aversive imagery and worrisome thinking. *Behavior Therapy, 24,* 457–466.

Lyubomirsky, S., King, L., & Diener, E. (2005). The benefits of frequent positive affect: Does happiness lead to success? *Psychological Bulletin, 131,* 803–855.

Lyubomirsky, S., & Lepper, H. S. (1999). A measure of subjective happiness: Preliminary reliability and construct validation. *Social Indicators Research, 46,* 137–155.

MacLeod, A. K., & Cropley, M. L. (1996). Anxiety, depression, and the anticipation of future positive and negative experiences. *Journal of Abnormal Psychology, 105,* 286–289.

Mandel, D. R., Hilton, D. J., & Catellani, P. (2005). *The psychology of counterfactual thinking.* London: Routledge.

Markus, H. R., & Kitayama, S. (1991). Culture and the self: Implications for cognition, emotion, and motivation. *Psychological Review, 98,* 224–253.

Marroquín, B. (2011). Interpersonal emotion regulation as a mechanism of social support in depression. *Clinical Psychology Review, 31,* 1276–1290.

Mayer, J. D., & Gaschke, Y. N. (1988). The experience and meta-experience of mood. *Journal of Personality and Social Psychology, 55,* 102–111.

Mayer, J. D., & Salovey, P. (1997). What is emotional intelligence? In P. Salovey & D. Sluyter (Eds.), *Emotional development and emotional intelligence: Educational implications* (pp. 3–31). New York: Basic Books.

Mayhew, S. L., & Gilbert, P. (2008). Compassionate mind training with people who hear malevolent voices: A case series report. *Clinical Psychology and Psychotherapy, 15,* 113–136.

Mayr, E. (1974). Behavior programs and evolutionary strategies. *American Scientist, 62,* 650–659.

McConnell, A. R., Niedermeier, K. E., Leibold, J. M., El-Alayli, A. G., Chin, P. P., & Kuipers, N. M. (2000). Someplace else? Role of prefactual thinking and anticipated regret in consumer behavior. *Psychology and Marketing, 17,* 281–298.

McNally, R. J. (2011). *What is mental illness?* Cambridge, MA: Belknap Press of Harvard University Press.

Mead, G. H. (1925). The genesis of the self and social control. *International Journal of Ethics, 35,* 251–273.

Mead, G. H. (1934). *Mind, self, and society.* Chicago: University of Chicago Press.

Melbourne Academic Mindfulness Interest Group. (2006). Mindfulness-based psychotherapies: A review of conceptual foundations, empirical evidence and practical considerations. *Australian and New Zealand Journal of Psychiatry, 40,* 285–294.

Mennin, D. S., Heimberg, R. G., Turk, C. L., & Fresco, D. M. (2005). Preliminary evidence for an emotion dysregulation model of generalized anxiety disorder. *Behaviour Research and Therapy, 43,* 1281–1310.

Menzulis, A. H., Abramson, L. Y., Hyde, J. S., & Hankin, B. L. (2004). Is there a universal positive bias in attributions?: A meta-analytic review of individual, developmental, and cultural difference in the self-serving attributional bias. *Psychological Bulletin, 130,* 711–747.

Meyer, T. J., Miller, M. L., Metzger, R. L., & Borkovec, T. D. (1990). Development and validation of the Penn State Worry Questionnaire. *Behaviour Research and Therapy, 28,* 487–495.

Mikulincer, M., & Shaver, P. R. (2007). *Attachment in adulthood: Structure, dynamics, and change.* New York: Guilford Press.

Mill, J. S. (2001). *Utilitarianism* (2nd ed.). Indianapolis, IN: Hackett. (Original work published 1861)

Mischel, W. (1979). On the interface of cognition and personality: Beyond the person–situation debate. *American Psychologist, 34,* 740–754.

Mischel, W., Shoda, Y., & Rodriguez, M. I. (1989) Delay of gratification in children. *Science, 244,* 933–938.

Moffitt, T. E., Arsenault, L., Belsky, D., Dickson, N., Hancox, R. J., Harrington, H., et al. (2011). A gradient of childhood self-control predicts health, wealth, and public safety. *Proceedings of the National Academy of Sciences, 108,* 2693–2698.

Moore, M. T., & Fresco, D. M. (2012). Depressive realism: A meta-analytic review. *Clinical Psychology Review, 32,* 496–509.

Mor, N., & Winquist, J. (2002). Self-focused attention and negative affect: A meta-analysis. *Psychological Bulletin, 128,* 638–662.

Morris, A. S., Silk, J. S., Steinberg, L., Myers, S. S., & Robinson, L. R. (2007). The role of the family context in the development of emotion regulation. *Social Development, 16,* 361–388.

Mowrer, O. H. (1960). *Learning theory and behavior.* New York: Wiley.

Murray, L., Creswell, C., & Cooper, P. J. (2009). The development of anxiety disorders in childhood: An integrative review. *Psychological Medicine, 39,* 1413–1423.

Myers, D. G. (2000). The funds, friends, and faith of happy people. *American Psychologist, 55,* 56–67.

Myers, D. G., & Diener, E. (1995). Who is happy? *Psychological Science, 6,* 10–19.

Neff, K. D. (2003). Self-compassion: An alternative conceptualization of a health attitude toward oneself. *Self and Identity, 2,* 85–101.

Neff, K. D., & Vonk, R. (2009). Self-compassion versus global self-esteem: Two different ways of relating to oneself. *Journal of Personality, 77,* 24–50.

Nemiah, J. C., Freyberger, H., & Sifneos, P. E. (1976). Alexithymia: A view of the psychosomatic process. In O. W. Hill (Ed.), *Modern trends in psychosomatic medicine* (Vol. 3, pp. 430–439). London: Butterworths.

Nitschke, J. B., & Heller, W. (2002). The neuropsychology of anxiety disorders: Affect, cognition, and neural circuitry. In H. D'haenen, J. A. den Boer, & P. Willner (Eds.), *Biological psychiatry* (pp. 975–988). New York: Wiley.

Nolen-Hoeksema, S. (2000). The role of rumination in depressive disorders and mixed anxiety/depressive symptoms. *Journal of Abnormal Psychology, 109,* 504–511.

Nolen-Hoeksema, S., & Davis, C. G. (1999). "Thanks for sharing that": Ruminators and their social support networks. *Journal of Personality and Social Psychology, 77,* 801–814.

Nolen-Hoeksema, S., Morrow, J., & Fredrickson, B. L. (1993). Response styles and the duration of episodes of depressed mood. *Journal of Abnormal Psychology, 102,* 20–28.

Nolen-Hoeksema, S., Wisco, B., & Lyubomirsky, S. (2008). Rethinking rumination. *Perspectives on Psychological Science, 3,* 400–424.

Ochsner, K. N., Bunge, S. A., Gross, J. J., & Gabrieli, J. D. (2002). Rethinking feelings: An fMRI study of the cognitive regulation of emotion. *Journal of Cognitive Neuroscience, 14,* 1215–1229.

Ochsner, K. N., & Gross, J. J. (2008). Cognitive emotion regulation: Insights from social cognitive and affective neuroscience. *Current Directions in Psychological Science, 17,* 153–158.

Olson, S. L., & Sameroff, A. J. (Ed.). (2009). *Biopsychosocial regulatory processes in the development of childhood behavioral problems.* New York: Cambridge University Press.

Ortony, A., & Turner, T. J. (1990). What's basic about basic emotions? *Psychological Review, 97,* 315–331.

Pace, T. W. W., Negi, L. T., Adame, D. D., Cole, S. P., Sivilli, T. I., Brown, T. D., et al. (2009). Effect of compassion meditation on neuroendocrine, innate immune and behavioral responses to psychosocial stress. *Psychoneuroendocrinology, 34,* 87–98.

Pace, T. W. W., Negi, L. T., Sivilli, T. I., Issa, M. J., Cole, S. P., Adame, D. D., et al. (2010). Innate immune, neuroendocrine and behavioral responses to psychosocial stress do not predict subsequent compassion meditation practice time. *Psychoneuroendocrinology, 35,* 310–315.

Pandita, S. U. (1992). *In this very life.* Boston: Wisdom.

Panksepp, J., & Biven, L. (2010). *The archaeology of mind: Neural origins of human emotions.* New York: Norton.

Pasch, L. A., Bradbury, T. N., & Davila, J. (1997). Gender, negative affectivity, and observed social support behavior in marital interaction. *Personal Relationships, 4,* 361–378.

Pennebaker, J. W. (1997). Writing about emotional experiences as a therapeutic process. *Psychological Science, 8,* 162–166.

Pezawas, L., Meyer-Lindenberg, A., Drabant, E. M., Verchinski, B. A., Munoz, K. E., Kolachana, B. S., et al. (2005). 5-HTTLPR polymorphism impacts human cingulate–amygdala interactions: A genetic susceptibility mechanism for depression. *Nature Neuroscience, 8,* 828–834.

Pfaffmann, C. (1960). The pleasures of sensation. *Psychological Review, 67,* 253–268.

Plutchik, R. (1980). *Emotion: A psychoevolutionary synthesis.* New York: Harper & Row.

Plutchik, R. (2000). *Emotions in the practice of psychotherapy: Clinical implications of affect theories.* Washington, DC: American Psychological Association Press.

Posner, J., Russell, J. A., & Peterson, B. S. (2005). The circumplex model of affect: An integrative approach to affective neuroscience, cognitive development, and psychopathology. *Development and Psychopathology, 17,* 715–734.

Posner, M. I., & Rothbart, M. K. (2000). Developing mechanisms of self-regulation. *Development and Psychopathology, 12,* 427–441.

Poulton, R., & Menzies, R.G. (2002). Non-associative fear acquisitions: A review of the evidence from retrospective and longitudinal research. *Behaviour Research and Therapy, 40,* 127–149.

Povinelli, D. J. (1995). The unduplicated self. In P. Rochat (Ed.), *The self in early infancy* (pp. 161–192). Amsterdam: North-Holland/Elsevier.

Preston, S. D., & de Waal, F. B. (2002). Empathy: Its ultimate and proximate bases. *Behavioural Brain Sciences, 25,* 1–20.

Pyszczynski, T., & Greenberg, J. (1987). Self-regulatory perseveration and the depressive self-focusing style: A self-awareness theory of reactive depression. *Psychological Bulletin, 102,* 122–138.

Quay, H. C. (1988). The behavioral reward and inhibition system in childhood behavior disorders. In L. M. Bloomingdale (Ed.), *Attention deficit disorder* (Vol. 3, pp. 176–186). Elmsford, NY: Pergamon Press.

Quay, H. C. (1993). The psychobiology of undersocialized aggressive conduct disorder: A theoretical perspective. *Development and Psychopathology, 5,* 165–180.

Raichle, M. E. (2006). The brain's dark energy. *Science, 314,* 1249–1250.

Raichle, M. E., MacLeod, A. M., Snyder, A. Z., Powers, W. J., Gusnard, D. A., & Shulman, G. L. (2001). A default mode of brain function. *Proceedings of the National Academy of Sciences of the USA, 98,* 676–682.

Rehman, U. S., Ginting, J., Karimiha, G., & Goodnight, J. A. (2010). Revisiting the relationship between depressive symptoms and marital communication using an experimental paradigm: The moderating effect of acute sad mood. *Behaviour Research and Therapy, 48,* 97–105.

Rehman, U. S., Gollan, J., & Mortimer, A. R. (2008). The marital context of depression: Research, limitations, and new directions. *Clinical Psychology Review, 28,* 179–198.

Remington, N., Fabrigar, L., & Visser, P. (2000). Reexamining the circumplex model of affect. *Journal of Personality and Social Psychology, 79,* 286–300.

Robinson, T. E., & Berridge, K. C. (2003). Addiction. *Annual Review of Psychology, 54,* 25–53.

Roese, N. J. (1997). Counterfactual thinking. *Psychological Bulletin, 121,* 133–134.

Rogers, C. R. (1951). *Client-centered therapy.* New York: Houghton Mifflin.

Rolls, E. T. (2005). *Emotion explained.* Oxford, UK: Oxford University Press.

Rolls, E. T. (2013). What are emotional states, and why do we have them? *Emotion Review, 5,* 241–247.

Rozanski, A., & Kubzansky, L. D. (2005). Psychologic functioning and physical health: A paradigm of flexibility. *Psychosomatic Medicine, 67,* S47–S53.

Ruby, P., & Decety, J. (2004). How would you feel versus how do you think she would feel?: A neuroimaging study of perspective-taking with social emotions. *Journal of Cognitive Neuroscience, 16,* 988–999.

Russell, J. A. (1980). A circumplex model of affect. *Journal of Personality and Social Psychology, 39,* 1161–1178.

Russell, J. A. (2003). Core affect and the psychological construction of emotion. *Psychological Review, 110,* 145–172.

Russell, J. A., & Barrett, L. F. (1999). Core affect, prototypical emotional episodes, and other things called emotion: Dissecting the elephant. *Journal of Personality and Social Psychology, 76,* 805–819.

Russell, J. A., & Carroll, J. M. (1999). On the bipolarity of positive and negative affect. *Psychological Bulletin, 125,* 3–30.

Ryan, R. M., & Deci, E. L. (2000). Self-determination theory and the facilitation of intrinsic motivation, social development, and well-being. *American Psychologist, 55,* 68–78.

Ryan, R. M., Kuhl, J., & Deci, E. L. (1997). Nature and autonomy: An organizational view of social and neurobiological aspects of self-regulation in behavior and development. *Development and Psychopathology, 9,* 701–728.

Salovey, P., & Mayer, J. D. (1990). Emotional intelligence. *Imagination, Cognition and Personality, 9,* 185–211.

Salovey, P., Mayer, J. D., Goldman, S. L., Turvey, C., & Palfai, T. P. (1995). Emotional attention, clarity, and repair: Exploring emotional intelligence using the Trait Meta-Mood Scale. In J. W. Pennebaker (Ed.), *Emotion, disclosure and health* (pp. 125–154). Washington, DC: American Psychological Association.

Salzberg, S. (1995). *Loving-kindness.* Boston: Shambhala.

Sarbin, T. R. (1952). A preface to a psychological analysis of the self. *Psychological Review, 59,* 11–22.

Schachter, S., & Singer, J. E. (1962). Cognitive, social, and physiological determinants of emotional state. *Psychological Review, 69*, 379–399.

Scherer, K. R., & Ellgring, H. (2007). Multimodal expression of emotion: Affect programs or componential appraisal patterns? *Emotion, 7*, 158–171.

Schultheiss, O. C., & Wirth, M. M. (2008). Biopsychological aspects of motivation. In J. Heckhausen & H. Heckhausen (Eds.), *Motivation and action* (2nd ed., pp. 247–271). New York: Cambridge University Press.

Schulz, S. M., Alpers, G. W., & Hofmann, S. G. (2008). Negative self-focused cognitions mediate the effect of trait social anxiety on state anxiety. *Behaviour Research and Therapy, 46*, 438–449.

Schutte, N. S., Malouff, J. M., Hall, L. E., Haggerty, D. J., Cooper, J. T., Golden, C. J., et al. (1998). Development and validation of a measure of emotional intelligence. *Personality and Individual Differences, 25*, 167–177.

Schwartz, C. E., Wright, C. L., Shin, L. M., Kagan, J., & Rauch, S. L. (2003). Inhibited and uninhibited infants "grown up": Adult amygdalar response to novelty. *Science, 300*, 1952–1953.

Schwartz, R. M. (1986). The internal dialogue: On the asymmetry between positive and negative coping thoughts. *Cognitive Therapy and Research, 10*, 591–605.

Schwartz, R. M. (1997). Consider the simple screw: Cognitive science, quality improvement, and psychotherapy. *Journal of Consulting and Clinical Psychology, 65*, 970–983.

Schwartz, R. M., & Garamoni, G. L. (1989). Cognitive balance and psychopathology: Evaluation of an information-processing model of positive and negative states of mind. *Clinical Psychological Review, 9*, 271–294.

Scitovsky, T. (1982). *The joyless economy.* New York: Oxford University Press.

Segal, Z. V., Williams, J. M. G., & Teasdale, J. D. (2002). *Mindfulness-based cognitive therapy for depression: A new approach to preventing relapse.* New York: Guilford Press.

Segerstrom, S. C., Stanton, A. L., Alden, L. E., & Shortridge, B. E. (2003). A multidimensional structure of repetitive thought: What's on your mind, and how, and how much? *Journal of Personality and Social Psychology, 85*, 909–921.

Seligman, M. E. P., & Csikszentmihalyi, M. (2000). Positive psychology: An introduction. *American Psychologist, 55*, 5–14.

Shafran, R., Thordarson, D., & Rachman, S. (1996). Thought–action fusion in obsessive compulsive disorder. *Journal of Anxiety Disorders, 10*, 379–391.

Sheng-Yen, M. (2001). *Hoofprints of the ox: Principles of the Chan Buddhist path as taught by a modern Chinese master.* New York: Oxford University Press.

Sheppes, G., Scheibe, S., Sutir, G., Radu, P., Blechert, J., & Gross, J. (2014).

Emotion regulation choice: A conceptual framework and supporting evidence. *Journal of Experimental Psychology: General, 143*, 163–181.

Silk, J. S., Steinberg, L., & Morris, A. S. (2005). Adolescents' emotion regulation in daily life: Links to depressive symptoms and problem behavior. *Child Development, 74*, 1869–1880.

Sloan, D. M., & Marx, B. P. (2004). A closer examination of the structured written disclosure procedure. *Journal of Consulting and Clinical Psychology, 72*, 165–175.

Snygg, D., & Combs, A. W. (1949). *Individual behavior.* New York: Harper & Row.

Solomon, R. L., & Corbit, J. D. (1974). An opponent-process theory of motivation: Temporal dynamics of affect. *Psychological Review, 81*, 119–145.

Solomon, R. L., & Wynne, L. C. (1953). Traumatic avoidance learning: Acquisition in normal dogs. *Psychological Monographs: General and Applied, 67*(4), 1–19.

Spence, K. W. (1956). *Behavior theory and conditioning.* New Haven, CT: Yale University Press.

Stice, E. (2002). Risk and maintenance factors for eating pathology: A meta-analytic review. *Psychological Bulletin, 128*, 825–848.

Stice, E., & Agras, W. S. (1999). Subtyping bulimic women along dietary restraint and negative affect dimensions. *Journal of Consulting and Clinical Psychology, 67*, 460–469.

Stice, E., Ragan, J., & Randall, P. (2004). Prospective relations between social support and depression: Differential direction of effects for parent and peer support? *Journal of Abnormal Psychology, 113*, 155–159.

Stöber, J., & Borkovec, T. D. (2002). Reduced concreteness of worry in generalized anxiety disorder: Findings from a therapy study. *Cognitive Therapy and Research, 26*, 89–96.

Suh, E., Diener, E., Oishi, S., & Triandis, H. C. (1998). The shifting basis of life satisfaction judgments across cultures: Emotions versus norms. *Journal of Personality and Social Psychology, 74*, 482–493.

Suvak, M. K., Litz, B. T., Sloan, D. M., Zanarini, M. C., Barrett, L. F., & Hofmann, S. G. (2011). Emotional granularity and borderline personality disorder. *Journal of Abnormal Psychology, 120*, 414–426.

Szasz, P. L., Szentagotai, A., & Hofmann, S. G. (2011). The effect of emotion regulation strategies on anger. *Behaviour Research and Therapy, 49*, 114–119.

Szasz, P. L., Szentagotai, A., & Hofmann, S. G. (2012). Effects of emotion regulation strategies on smoking craving, attentional bias, and task persistence. *Behaviour Research and Therapy, 50*, 333–340.

Szasz, T. (1961). *The myth of mental illness: Foundations of a theory of personal conduct.* New York: Hoeber-Harper.

Taylor, G. J., Bagby, R. M., & Parker, J. D. A. (1997). *Disorders of affect regulation: Alexithymia in medical and psychiatric illness.* Cambridge, UK: Cambridge University Press.

Terracciano, A., McCrae, R., Hagemann, D., & Costa, P. (2003). Individual difference variables, affective differentiation, and the structures of affect. *Journal of Personality, 71,* 669–703.

Thayer, J. F., Friedman, B. H., & Borkovec, T. D. (1996). Autonomic characteristics of generalized anxiety disorder and worry. *Biological Psychiatry, 39,* 255–266.

Toates, F. (1986). *Motivational systems.* New York: Cambridge University Press.

Tomkins, S. S. (1963). *Affect, imagery, consciousness: Vol. 2. The negative affects.* New York: Springer.

Tomkins, S. S. (1982). Affect theory. In P. Ekman (Ed.), *Emotion in the human face* (2nd ed., pp. 353–395). Cambridge, UK: Cambridge University Press.

Travis, L., Lyness, J. M., Shields, C. G., King, D. A., & Cox, C. (2004). Social support, depression, and functional disability in older adult primary-care patients. *American Journal of Geriatric Psychiatry, 12,* 265–271.

Treynor, W., Gonzalez, R., & Nolen-Hoeksema, S. (2003). Rumination reconsidered: A psychometric analysis. *Cognitive Therapy and Research, 27,* 247–259.

Tucker, D. M., & Newman, J. P. (1981). Verbal versus imaginal cognitive strategies in the inhibition of emotional arousal. *Cognitive Therapy and Research, 5,* 197–202.

Van Boven, L., & Loewenstein, G. (2003). Social projection of transient drive states. *Personality and Social Psychology Bulletin, 29,* 1159–1168.

van Strien, T., Engels, R. C. M. E., Leeuwe, J. V., & Snoek, H. M. (2005). The Stice model of overeating: Tests in clinical and non-clinical samples. *Appetite, 45,* 205–213.

Vitaliano, P. P., DeWolfe, D. J., Mairuro, R. D., Russo, J., & Katon, W. (1990). Appraisal changeability of a stressor as a modifier of the relationship between coping and depression: A test of the hypothesis of fit. *Journal of Personality and Social Psychology, 59,* 582–592.

Vrana, S. R., Cuthbert, B. N., & Lang, P. J. (1986). Fear imagery and text processing. *Psychophysiology, 23,* 247–253.

Wakefield, J. C. (2007). The concept of mental disorder: Diagnostic implications of the harmful dysfunction analysis. *World Psychiatry, 6,* 149–156.

Watkins, E. (2004). Appraisals and strategies associated with rumination and worry. *Personality and Individual Differences, 37,* 679–694.

Watson, D., Clark, L. A., & Tellegen, A. (1988). Development and validation of brief measure of positive and negative affect: The PANAS scales. *Journal of Personality and Social Psychology 54,* 1063–1070.

Watson, D., Wiese, D., Vaidya, J., & Tellegen, A. (1999). The two general activation systems of affect: Structural findings, evolutionary considerations, and psychobiological evidence. *Journal of Personality and Social Psychology, 76,* 820–838.

Wegner, D. M., Schneider, D. J., Carter, S. R., & White, T. L. (1987). Paradoxical effects of thought suppression. *Journal of Personality and Social Psychology, 52,* 5–13.

Wegner, D. M., & Zanakos, S. (1994). Chronic thought suppression. *Journal of Personality, 62,* 615–640.

Wells, A., & Papageorgiou, C. (1998). Social phobia: Effects of external attention on anxiety, negative beliefs, and perspective taking. *Behavior Therapy, 29,* 357–370.

White, J. L., Moffitt, T. E., Caspi, A., Bartusch, D. J., Needles, D. J., & Stouthamer-Loeber, M. (1994). Measuring impulsivity and examining its relationship to delinquency. *Journal of Abnormal Psychology, 103,* 192–205.

Williams, M., & Penman, D. (2011). *Mindfulness: An eight-week plan for finding peace in a frantic world.* New York: Rodale Books.

Wilson, T. D., Wheatley, T. P., Meyers, J. M., Gilbert, D. T., & Axsom, D. (2000). Focalism: A source of durability bias in affective forecasting. *Journal of Personality and Social Psychology, 78,* 821–836.

Winter, K. A., & Kuiper, N. A. (1997). Individual differences in the experience of emotions. *Clinical Psychology Review, 17,* 791–821.

Wirtz, C. M., Hofmann, S. G., Riper, H., & Berking, M. (2014). Emotion regulation predicts anxiety over a five-year interval: A cross-lagged panel analysis. *Depression and Anxiety, 31,* 87–95.

Yap, M. B. H., Allen, N. B., & Ladouceur, C. D. (2008). Maternal socialization of positive affect: The impact of invalidation on adolescent emotion regulation and depressive symptomatology. *Child Development, 79,* 1415–1431.

Yik, M., Russell, J. A., & Steiger, J. H. (2011). A 12-point circumplex structure of core affect. *Emotion, 11,* 705–731.

Young, J. E., Klosko, J. S., & Weishaar, M. E. (2003). *Schema therapy: A practitioner's guide.* New York: Guilford Press.

Young, P. T. (1966). Hedonic organization and regulation of behavior. *Psychological Review, 73,* 59–86.

Zaki, J., & Williams, W. C. (2013). Interpersonal emotion regulation. *Emotion, 13,* 803–810.

Index

Note: f following a page number indicates a figure or a table.